# The Weight Maintenance Manual

## how to achieve and maintain your ideal weight

Steve Marshall
and Caroline Ross

*From Steve to Ann,*
*who kept me on the straight and narrow*

*From Caroline to Pamela, Charles, Jethro, and Olivia:*
*may you never need it!*

# About the Authors

Our backgrounds are quite different – Steve has dealt mainly with numbers and Caroline mainly with people. We both have day jobs, with Steve enjoying a second career as a musician. We have both had a lot of experience of teaching and of writing. Unfortunately, we have both also had a lot of experience of alternating between losing weight and gaining weight. What kept getting in the way, as we finally found out, was that losing weight is one thing, but keeping it off is another thing altogether.

This is the book we wish we had been able to read before we started our first diets. But we have talked about this, and we are pretty convinced that even if such a book had existed, we wouldn't have read it! After all, we were both intelligent people with a reasonable understanding of food and nutrition. How hard could losing weight be? What could go wrong? We found out that the answers were 'very' and 'plenty'.

We were fortunate – we discovered a weight-loss website and app called *Nutracheck*, we slimmed down to healthy target weights, and we have since maintained our weight at those targets. And somewhere along that often-rocky maintenance road, we got to know one another on a discussion forum. We helped one another, met up 'in real life', and we are now both one another's diet coach (we'll explain that later) and also firm friends. And we are still firm friends, despite the stresses of writing a book together!

We think it may be interesting to give you an overview here of our weight over the years and the problems we came up against. We certainly have found that we are more inclined to take notice of what someone says about weight loss if the person saying it has had problems themselves.

## Something about my weight history, by Steve

I come from a family where many people are overweight. I was a large (eleven-pound) baby with a big appetite, and for the next twenty years I was always on a diet, and I was nearly always overweight – a textbook expert dieter but hopeless maintainer. I lost a few stone when I started work, but the weight gradually crept back on (with a bit more for luck), and that set the 'yo-yo' trend for the next forty years.

At the age of sixty-one I weighed 23 st 6 lb, a high and dangerous weight, even for my 6' 1" frame. I was pre-diabetic, I had high blood pressure, and I could hardly walk.

I joined *Nutracheck* and, from somewhere, I discovered some powerful motivation, as well as a method of weight loss that suited me. In twenty months, I slimmed down to 13 st 2 lb, and in the several years since then, I have maintained my weight loss. That's not to say it has been easy – I have seen some significant weight fluctuations (up *and* down) – but I am still at my target weight, which is a healthy weight for my height.

**Something about my weight history, by Caroline**
I was a plump baby and toddler but not a particularly fat child. I recall standing on the scales, aged twenty-one and 5' 4", weighing just over nine stone. I didn't weigh regularly, so clearly I wasn't thinking much about my weight, but my clothes size drifted up over the years, and the next weight-related memory I have is when I was twenty-eight, wanted to lose some weight, and got down to a size 12–14 by using diet milkshakes. I got a bit fed up with that, went back to 'normal eating', and my clothes size went to 14–16 and stayed there for several years.

In my mid-thirties, I gave birth at around ten stone. Then the trouble started, when I ate rather too much, and too much of the wrong things, while on maternity leave. I never managed to lose that weight, and four years later, I was thirteen stone and 'moderately obese'. Then followed ten years of weight loss/weight gain/repeat ('yo-yo dieting').

In desperation, I decided to simply count calories, and I stumbled across *Nutracheck* on the internet. Early on, I read a blog by one Steve Marshall, and so began a connection that has helped me reduce my weight to a healthy nine stone and, with some wobbles, maintain that weight.

# Table of Contents

**PART 3**
**What you need to understand**
**so you can maintain your target weight forever**

**PART 4**
**The actions that you need to take**
**so you can maintain your target weight forever**

# Preamble

## PLEASE READ THIS FIRST!

**Even if you don't usually read introductions, prologues, preambles, or anything of that sort, please make an exception here. It's not long, and we have packed it full of useful information about how the book works and how to get the most out of it. Here we go ...**

## Welcome!

Hello, we are Steve and Caroline. Welcome to our book. Now here is the traditional dramatic statement, designed to persuade you to buy this book, if you haven't already:

**Between the two of us, we lost fifteen stone, and we have kept it off for several years. This book tells you how we did it, and it will help you to do it too.**

Looks good! But we are honourable people, and we now want to tell you our top six basic beliefs about weight loss and maintenance. If you don't share at least most of these basic beliefs, our book may not be for you, and you may prefer to spend your hard-earned money on something else. Our basic beliefs are:

• Although losing weight is important, what *really* matters is maintaining that weight loss in the long term.

• There is only one way to lose weight – that is to consume fewer calories than your body burns. (With the exception of a very few people with certain medical conditions.)

• It is crucial to find a way of limiting calories consumed. There are different ways of doing that, but we believe that the most effective, simple, reliable, and flexible way of limiting calories – by far – is to count those calories.

• Exercise is useful because it increases calories burned, but, for weight loss and for most people, it is nowhere near as useful as limiting calories consumed.

• It is important to weigh yourself regularly.

• A sound approach is to follow current scientific thinking, backed by the best evidence. If we are in doubt about which thinking that is, we go with NHS-based information rather than information from a nutritionist/diet guru who is the latest big thing on the TV or the internet.

We will explain these points in detail, but we wanted to give you the headlines now, so you know what sort of book you are looking at. It is not a book that pushes exciting and exotic new miracle diets – diets that, somehow, the entire medical establishment has been too stupid to notice until now! It is a book that clearly explains how to lose weight and how to keep it off using simple, non-fad techniques.

**Why do we think we will be able to help you?**
We hope that you are still with us! Although on second thoughts, you may be wondering why you should take any notice of this book when there are many thousands of books on the subject of dieting, and some of them by household names in the dieting game. Almost certainly you have never heard of Steve Marshall or Caroline Ross, so why can *they* help you?

We think we are in a good position to help you because both of us lost large amounts of weight, and have kept it off for a long time, by using a clear, practical, and fad-free method. All the signs so far are that this is going to be our final diet – the one that works forever. Although nothing is guaranteed about the human body, if you follow our book closely and keep everything simple, we would be surprised indeed if this diet is not *your* final diet as well.

But it is not going to be dead easy. We can't do it for you. There is no alternative to changing what you eat and changing the way you think about food – after all, if you didn't need to change these, you probably wouldn't need to lose weight in the first place. There is no secret, special pill or magic formula. If you are not prepared to change what you eat and the way you think about food, this is probably not the book for you. You might need it, but you won't use it. So if you are not prepared to make changes, we suggest you put the book down and move away.

**Who did we write this book for?**
Pretty obviously, given what we said above about our basic beliefs, we wrote this book for people who have similar basic beliefs to ours about weight loss and maintenance. We know that there are other ways of trying to lose weight, and we know a little about them, but it is

controlling calories and weighing regularly that have worked for us, and this book is based on doing those things. But if you are still reading, we think that you will benefit from the book, whatever your history of body weight:

• If you come to this book as you begin your first-ever weight loss – **welcome, this book was written for you!**
• If you come to this book having lost weight and wanting to maintain – **welcome, this book was written for you!**
• If you come to this book having (like ourselves) lost and regained weight, maybe several times – **welcome, this book was written for you!**

Whatever your dieting history (or wherever you are currently in the weight loss/weight gain/repeat cycle), this book can help you because it is based on the idea that long-term maintenance of a healthy weight depends on losing weight in a way that you will be able to stick to for a long time. The word for such a way is 'sustainable' – a word you will come across again in this book.

Our book is therefore about sustainable weight loss (and overcoming the barriers to this) and also about how you can move into a lifetime of maintenance of your new weight.

Because of our approach, we think you will find plenty of ideas and tips that will help you to become one of the elite group of people who lose weight and keep it off. Whether it is the first or the thirty-first diet you have been on, we can help you make it the last one!

### What the book is (and isn't)

This book helps you to understand what is important in the business of losing weight and maintaining your target weight in the long term. It also gives guidance about what you might do in order to achieve that weight loss and weight maintenance. But success will be easier and more likely if you understand what the book is:

• It is not a diet book, promoting one particular diet. We suggest broad healthy eating principles, but the details of your diet will be up to you. In fact, many details of the diets of Steve and Caroline are different, although many are similar.
• It is not a prescriptive diet plan, although there are some elements that we believe are common to any successful weight loss plan, and we emphasise those.
• It is not a book of recipes, although we do give a few general-purpose thoughts about food preparation that have served us well.

• It is not a simple and magic solution to your dieting problems. Make no mistake, there is no effortless way of maintaining your weight loss (or losing weight in the first place).

## What is special about this book?

You may have noticed that books about dieting are heavily focused on losing weight and achieving a target weight. They rarely touch on what happens next, and if they do, the advice is almost always brief. In fact, we cannot remember ever seeing another book that *focuses* on weight maintenance. That's a big pity, because the statistics (and everyone we have spoken to on the subject) suggest that maintaining target weight is extremely difficult and that most people fail – sooner or later. Maintaining target weight is what people seem to need most help with, but that is the very help that they don't get.

Our book, unusually among 'diet books', therefore has a big emphasis on maintaining your target weight forever. If you are reading this, it is unlikely that this is your first-ever diet. Even if you have successfully lost weight in the past, you may well have regained some or all of it – many, many people do. We both lost weight several times before but never kept it off for a long time. Until recently. We have therefore written this book to share with you our approach to losing weight, which makes keeping it off forever much more likely. And that is why our book is so called – it is Steve and Caroline's *Weight Maintenance Manual*.

We think that there is something else that makes the *Weight Maintenance Manual* special, and that is that we have split it into four parts. We are aware that splitting it in this way is unusual, so we'll just spend a little time to explain why we have done it like that. The underlying reason is that we are convinced that it is nearly impossible to maintain target weight forever (or even for a few years) unless achieving that target weight was done in the right way. Achieving that target weight in the right way is difficult unless the right foundations are laid down at the very start. So the book is split the way it is in order to give you the best chance of succeeding now – and far into the future.

• **Part 1** is about what you need to *understand* in order to make our whole approach to weight loss work for you, so you lose weight successfully. All too often, people just launch themselves into a weight-loss diet without understanding how to approach it, and the diet fails.
• **Part 2** is about what you need to *do* in order to lose weight successfully, so you can arrive at the weight you want to be.

- **Part 3** is about further matters you need to *understand* to maintain that target weight forever. Armed with that understanding ...
- **Part 4** is about what you actually need to *do* in order to maintain your target weight in the long term.

### How to use this book

You can use this book in various ways:

- If you come to this book as you begin your first-ever diet, you will probably want to read it like a novel – part 1, then part 2. Later, when you are approaching your target weight, read parts 3 and 4.
- If you come to this book having lost weight and wanting to maintain, you will probably want to read parts 3 and 4. But if you lost your weight quickly on (for example) a very low-calorie diet, we suggest you begin with parts 1 and 2.
- If you come to this book having lost and regained weight, maybe several times (like we did), we strongly suggest that you begin with parts 1 and 2. That's because before you can make real progress, you will need to break the habits that caused that weight loss/weight gain/repeat cycle. Parts 1 and 2 will help you to do that. You can move on to parts 3 and 4 later.

You may also want to dip into the book because you have a specific problem with dieting. We have tried to make it easy for you to do that by dividing the book into a lot of chapters ('slices', as we've called them) and giving them clear and meaningful titles. Here are some examples:

- You know roughly what to do, but you just can't keep to it. You need motivation, and so slice 3 ('Get motivated and stay motivated') will appeal.
- You don't know how to diet. In that case, you need to understand about calories, and so slice 8 ('Understand the benefits of counting and recording calories') may catch your eye.
- Your previous diets have always been derailed by lots of social activities. You will probably find lots to interest you in slice 10 ('Decide on your approach to social eating events').

The book supports these and many other approaches because it is easy to find your way around it. The slice titles are meaningful, and the book tells a clear beginning-to-end story. You'll quickly get the hang of it.

Thank you for reading the Preamble. We think that's all we can usefully do to set the scene. So take a deep breath, carry on reading, and begin to discover our thoughts and advice on weight loss and weight maintenance!

## The Weight Maintenance Manual
### how to achieve and maintain
### your ideal weight

The four parts of The Weight Maintenance Manual are:

Part 1: What you need to understand
so you can lose weight successfully

Part 2: The actions that you need to take
so you can reach your target weight

Part 3: What you need to understand
so you can maintain your target weight forever

Part 4: The actions that you need to take
so you can maintain your target weight forever

# Welcome to

# Part 1

# What you need
# to understand
# so you can lose
# weight successfully

# Slice 1

# Understand why weight loss is so difficult

This first slice describes the difficulties there are in losing weight, but then it gives you the happy news that we can help you through those difficulties. The slice gives an introduction to what you need to do to succeed, and it points you to the right parts of the book for all the details.

**Why is it important to understand that losing weight is difficult?**
The rule for losing weight is simple and well known – eat less and move more. And yet few people find that losing weight is easy, and there is a lot of research evidence that tells us that, of those who manage to lose a substantial amount of weight, only a very small percentage keep it off, even for one year. We can back this up with our own experience – and probably you can too!

So it is strange that so many diet books, apps, websites, and organisations cheerfully (if inaccurately) tell you that with *their* approach to losing weight, it's easy. Or even that you can 'lose weight without dieting'. If any such claim were true, wouldn't we all be slim?

Human beings are complicated creatures, and those massive brains of ours mean that the way we think about and understand things makes a big difference to what we do. If you think something is going to be easy and then you find it difficult, it increases the chances that you will get fed up and give up. You are more likely to think along these lines: 'If the experts say it is easy and I find it so hard, then perhaps I'll never manage it. I might as well give up.' On the other hand, if you know it is tricky (but possible), it is more likely you will think: 'Hmmm, this bit isn't working well; what can I do to make it work?' Or we hope you might think: 'What do Steve and Caroline have to say about this?'

We believe forewarned is forearmed; if you know it is tricky to lose weight, you can manage the difficulties without giving up. When you understand that losing weight is not easy, you can treat yourself more kindly when you slip up and praise yourself when you make a wise choice. All of which makes it more likely you will persevere and not get fed up and give up.

Our experience is that losing weight is difficult but also that it *is* possible. Most people are repeat dieters – you have probably lost some weight before, so you *know* you can do it. The tricky part is keeping on doing it until you have got to a healthy weight and then maintaining that weight forever. We don't think there is anything special about us – we don't have amazing willpower, and we sometimes struggle to keep our weight where we want it to be, but, by and large, we manage. However, we never make the mistake of thinking it should be easy. That way, when it gets tough, we don't believe we are failing, and we're not tempted to give up – we just know we need to think about what is happening and how to make it work again.

## Why is weight loss so difficult?

We have already said that losing weight is a big project. It's easy to play at it, lose a few pounds, and then put all those pounds back on again. We are not interested in helping you to do that! Our book is all about losing weight and then keeping it off. And that *is* difficult, which is precisely why so few people manage to do it. The question then is 'Why is it difficult?' and the answer is in seven parts, which form the rest of this slice.

## Evolution makes losing weight difficult

Of the seven parts, some are likely to be more important for you than others. But this first one probably affects all of us in some way or another.

Being overweight is bad for your health in the long term, but it kills you slowly. Starvation kills much more quickly. So those of our remote ancestors who tended to put on weight were more likely to survive long enough to have children, and those children were likely to inherit the tendency, so they were also more likely to survive. And so on. The long-term problems of weight gain didn't matter much if you were likely to die of diseases, childbirth, or being savaged by a wild animal before you were forty.

Thousands of years later, many of us have inherited what used to be the useful tendency to put on weight, but now that tendency is no longer useful! The ancient problems of diseases, childbirth, or wild animals are much less common, and we live long enough (often to eighty or more) to suffer from modern killers. These are killers such as cancer, diabetes, strokes, and heart attacks – and they become more dangerous with the long-term problems of being overweight.

When there might not be enough food, the safest plan is to eat as much as you can because you never know where the next meal is going to come from. This made sense when we had to go out and hunt and gather our food, and days or weeks might go by without fresh foods being available. Nowadays we can easily get food within minutes because supermarkets have long opening hours. And you no longer even need to leave your house to get a takeaway meal – you can have it brought to your door. But the instinct to eat enough to ensure we are not hungry tomorrow, even if we will be eating again today, seems to still be there in many of us. Remember you are not a cave dweller, and there is plenty of food available. You can store leftovers in the fridge – you don't need to eat them!

Another evolutionary safety tactic is to prefer familiar foods because if you've had something before, you know it won't be poisonous. This also could be where the widespread liking of sweet foods comes from – because sweet things are rarely poisonous. In part 2 of the book, we encourage you to try new foods, but some people find that difficult. For them, it will be particularly important to gently point out that they are not cave dwellers, that many people have tried these foods before, and that they are safe!

## Our brains make losing weight difficult
Our brains are good at establishing habits, which is explained further in slice 2. Given a choice between doing something you have always done and doing something different, it is usually easiest to do what you have always done. The problem for weight loss comes when the habit is not a helpful one. And that is one big reason that it's difficult to lose weight – because your brain finds it hard to break habits (even bad ones). In fact, it is often easier to build up a new habit than try to break an old one.

Our brains also work against us when it comes to sweet foods. As we said above, we are programmed to like sweet (i.e. safe-to-eat) foods; furthermore, the parts of the brain connected with pleasure fire off when we eat sweet foods, which encourages us to eat them. Given that sweet foods are usually high in calories, this is not helpful when trying to lose weight!

## Our emotions make losing weight difficult
Many people use food as a way of managing emotions. This can become abundantly clear when you try to change your eating patterns to lose weight. We have four whole slices on emotional eating – it is an important reason why dieting can be difficult for some people.

99.9 per cent of dieters are going to slip up at some point and have a single meal or a whole day (or even longer) when they eat more than they intended. We need to find ways of managing any disappointment without giving up (slice 26 looks at this). Another disappointment can come when you have 'done everything right' for a few days, or even for a couple of weeks, but your weight is resolutely staying the same or even going up. This can make the faint-hearted dieter give up, but knowing this can happen helps you stick with the diet until your weight begins to drop again (see slice 25 for help with that).

**Time pressures can make losing weight difficult**
You will see as you read this book that some changes that you will need to make require time – sometimes quite a lot of time (when trying to increase exercise, for example). If you already have a busy life, making changes that are going to use up more of your precious time can be hard. We cover this later, in slice 6.

We will see (in slice 12) how time pressures can be eased while still doing what you need to do to lose weight. You can do that by thinking through how to make the time spent on your weight loss as short as it can be, focusing on activities you like doing or that you can see are really going to help you to lose weight. This will make your choices easier.

Changing what you eat, and therefore how you shop, cook, and manage leftover food, needs some thought and time – especially at first. Monitoring what you eat and what you weigh, wherever and however you do this, also takes some time. And planning and cooking your food may take even longer. Sometimes, and unfortunately, it is just easier to slip back into your old practices. Several slices in the book (including 6, 15, 16, and 18) will help with this.

To put it bluntly, these new diet-related drains on your time *should be* things that are so useful to your diet that you are happy to ease aside other activities. If you're *not* happy to do that, then maybe weight loss is not for you at the moment. Perhaps, in the future, losing weight will become a higher priority in your life, and then you can come back to us – we'll always be here!

**Choosing an inappropriate diet can make losing weight difficult**
People attempt to lose weight in many different ways, and every diet has people who swear by it. But whichever system you choose, it is important to be able to stick to it, possibly for a long time. The question to ask yourself is 'Is it – honestly – sustainable for me?' If you try to lose weight in a way that is – for you – too restrictive, too boring, too expensive, or even too complicated, it will probably drain your motivation more quickly. You will get fed up and give up.

Both of us, and many people we know, have tried a lot of different diets over the years, following each one for a time, until we get fed up and give up. The trick is to know what you will, really and truly, be able to live with for a long time. Slices 6 and 16 will help you with this one.

**Other people can make losing weight difficult**
There are many ways in which even our nearest and dearest can make weight loss more difficult. If they do not join you in your diet, then you may find yourself cooking different meals at the same time. If they don't want you to lose weight, for whatever reason, they might undermine your attempts by bringing you 'treats' to eat or drink. And how are you going to lose weight when others in the household like chocolate biscuits and leave them lying around to tempt you? Are you always going to put your diet second to what those nearest and dearest want to eat? How will you choose where you compromise?

Finally, even if your family and friends are exceptionally supportive in every way, there will be birthdays and events to celebrate with meals. We have a lot more to say about managing all of these difficulties in slice 22.

**The diet industry can make losing weight difficult**
We have fairly strong feelings on this subject, so it's a good time to introduce you to the book's 'chat time' idea. We use chat time when the best way to get our thoughts over to you is to write down a conversation we had. Often, like the one below, it was between Steve and Caroline, but sometimes we involved somebody else (maybe someone who had a particular problem we could help with). Here's the first one.

*CHAT TIME*

*CAROLINE: Have you noticed that as well as seeing a lot of 'losing weight is easy if you do it this way' media messages, there is also no shortage of 'diets don't work' messages?*

*STEVE: Yes. 'Do it this way' is an obvious selling job because 'the way' that is being promoted is usually to the benefit of the people doing the promoting. 'Diets don't work' is no more than another selling job – just a less obvious one!*

*CAROLINE: It's an unhelpful idea, which leads people to give up before they start. I suppose it comes from the fact that while a lot of people have temporarily lost weight while dieting, the evidence is that they put it back on again. And that's true, because a lot of the world is getting fatter and is suffering more weight-related illnesses.*

*STEVE: But, in a funny way, that huge diet industry doesn't mind if people believe that diets don't work, get demotivated, and give up. There's always another diet just around the corner for them to try. What the diet industry doesn't want is for us all to carefully follow a diet we believe in and all end up at a good weight. There would be no more need to diet, which would be bad for the diet industry – and repeat business is good business!*

*CAROLINE: But we know (including from our own experience) that most overweight people have lost weight at some point in their lives, even if they put it back on again. So diets do work – it's the maintenance of the weight loss that lets people down.*

*STEVE: This is where the idea of a 'lifestyle change' comes in.*

*CAROLINE: Yes! Diets don't work if you diet and then go back to your old eating patterns. But they do work if you make them a part of a new lifestyle.*

We are not usually people who like to 'rant', but the food industry is unhelpful to the dieter in various ways, and we all have to be alert to that fact. Some examples of this (but there are many more):
• Food labelling that calls calories 'energy' (as in 'energy drinks').
• Using small print that shows that a packet contains two portions when most people would assume it was a single portion.
• Branding food such as avocados or nuts as 'healthy fats', which may be true but skates over the fact that they are also high in calories.
• Describing products as 'low-fat' when the reduction of fat has been achieved by increasing the amount of sugar.

Be on your guard!

## Conclusion
All of the seven difficulties above are real, and yet **none of them has to stop you from losing weight and maintaining that weight loss**. We have faced those difficulties ourselves and, like all successful dieters, we

have had to find ways to overcome them. The rest of our book is about the ways we found to overcome those (and other) difficulties.

We said near the start of this slice that forewarned is forearmed. We hope that you now are.

In the end, it's up to you. But if you *really* want to lose weight, reach your healthy weight, and maintain that weight forever, then, with the help of this book, you will be able to.

# Slice 2

# Understand why you have to start acquiring good habits at the very beginning

Losing weight and keeping it off is more or less impossible without changing some of your habits. Changing those habits is what people mean when they say 'It's not a diet, it's a lifestyle change.' The bad news, however, is that calling your diet 'a lifestyle change' is not going to make much difference unless you actually *do change* your lifestyle as well. If you don't change your habits for the better, your weight control might succeed for a time, but in the longer term, you are more likely to fail. That is why we often discuss habits in this book – in fact, if you care to count them, we use the word 'habit' over 120 times!

We need to explain in some detail what this frequently used word means, because the determined weight loss maintainer needs to know something about habits and how they are formed. Knowing how to harness the power of habits rather than be ruled by them is useful! Once you have an understanding of habits under your belt, we think that you will find this book even more helpful in your weight loss and weight maintenance.

## What are habits and why do they matter?
To understand this, we need to understand a little about how our brains work. Think of your brain as a series of paths, which occasionally divide in two at a fork. If every time you come to a fork, you take the left-hand path, it will become well worn, easier to walk along, and more distinct. At the same time, the right-hand path – the one you never take – will get more overgrown and, in the end, might even disappear altogether as the brambles and nettles close in. If one day you do think about taking that right-hand path, you might not even be sure where the path is. And if you do spot it, it looks like hard work to walk along. If you are in a hurry or not wearing long trousers to protect you, it might just be easier to turn around and take the familiar left-hand path – again.

Taking a familiar path is what a habit is. Every time you do something by taking a particular path, your brain smooths out the path for you to make it easier to do it again. Let's look at some chat time, illustrating how this science can affect our everyday lives.

## CHAT TIME

STEVE: *I understand a little about why it's hard to break a habit such as having a big cheese sandwich when I am fed up and tired. It's all to do with these paths in my brain.*

CAROLINE: *Yes indeed. And I suppose that you have gone down that have-a-big-cheese-sandwich path quite often in your life.*

STEVE: *Err, yes. Very often.*

CAROLINE: *What that means is that the have-a-big-cheese-sandwich path in your brain is well used and will be an easy path to walk down next time. Well-used paths are easy to spot and convenient to take.*

STEVE: *I see that, but how do those paths become well used? I can understand a path can be used once, but what is it that makes us walk down a path for the second time?*

CAROLINE: *It seems to be about instant gratification versus long-term gain. Eating or drinking something that is immediately rewarding (because it tastes nice or gives you an immediate energy boost or relaxes you) is far more likely to be a path that we walk again. Before you know it, your brain will have it all worked out – 'Last time I went down that path, it was nice, so I'll do it again.' And there you are, tramping down any new growth on the have-a-big-cheese-sandwich path – and making it even clearer.*

STEVE: *So I guess that a behaviour that is not immediately rewarding won't be used much, even if it is beneficial to you in the long term. For example, a behaviour such as not having a big cheese sandwich is certainly not immediately rewarding! It's amazing we ever manage to change our habits at all.*

CAROLINE: *Fortunately, we are reasonably intelligent human beings, with free will and strong motivation to slim down to a healthy weight! It's that motivation that helps us to deliberately keep walking down an overgrown path. In the end, to use our example, the don't-have-a-big-cheese-sandwich path becomes clear and easy to walk down.*

*STEVE: It does sound like hard work. Is there a way to make treading a new path for oneself any easier or quicker?*

*CAROLINE: Luckily, there are a couple of ways. One way is to plan your route before you go – if you are determined that you are going to go down a new path, it helps you not be distracted by the other one, even if it is clear and inviting. The other way is if you give yourself a reward.*

*STEVE: What kind of a reward? Somehow I feel you aren't going to say a big cheese sandwich.*

*CAROLINE: Certainly not! You are already above having ideas like that. I mean a mental pat on the back, such as giving yourself an acknowledgement that you have made a good choice. Or you could tell a friend about your choice of the new path – a friend who knows how important doing that is to you, and who will be pleased to congratulate you. Or you could even put 10 pence in a savings pot. Anything except a food or drink reward!*

[From now on in the book, we will usually use 'food' to mean 'food and drink'.]

*STEVE: You mean I make it slightly easier to avoid having a big cheese sandwich tomorrow just by telling myself I've done well to avoid having a big cheese sandwich today.*

*CAROLINE: That's it. That good don't-have-a-big-cheese-sandwich path will have just become a little more familiar. And the more frequently and enthusiastically you choose it, the more the good path will become the one you follow automatically. When that happens, dieting is easier!*

Now we are all set to understand more about dieting and maintaining. Let's begin by looking at why it is so useful to acquire new habits at the start of your diet.

**Why you have to start acquiring new habits at the beginning of your diet**

To understand this, we are going to start by assuming that your old dieting habits have not worked well for you. To be blunt, if your old habits had worked well, you would not be overweight again now and you would not be reading this book. But don't feel bad – a great many people are in the same boat and have never been able to get out of that boat. *You will be able to* – as we both have. Read on!

Remember that your brain is always ready to help you to go down the same old paths. If you resent dieting and think of it as something to be done quickly so 'normal eating' can resume as soon as possible, then the new, helpful, and sustainable habits won't get built up in the same way. If you do not build up these new habits, you are less likely to reach your target weight, and even if you do, you are more likely to put the weight back on again. And then you will have to start all over again – and again and again! That is the dreaded, common, and obviously-named yo-yo dieting.

If, however, you see managing your weight in the long term as an exciting challenge that proves you are resourceful, determined, (and pretty clever), then it makes creating new habits an easier choice. Which in turn makes those new paths more inviting and means you are more likely to keep walking down them until the other paths grow over from disuse.

As we have already made clear, the whole point of this book is to help you to maintain your target body weight for good. Hence we are not interested in one-off short-term fixes and we are not interested in settling for yo-yo dieting. If you want to keep the weight off forever, the best way is – early on in your diet – to start making new habits that will make this possible and which you will be happy to follow for the rest of your life. You may not have noticed it, but that is what the shape of the line on the cover of the book intends to reflect.

The word often used for habits that can be followed for a long time is 'sustainable'. Such habits are pure gold because
• if you adopt good sustainable habits at the start of your diet, then
• you will still be following the habits when you hit your target weight, and
• that will give you a head start when you go into maintenance, and
• that will mean you have substantially increased your chances of being in the small minority of people who lose weight and keep it off, and
**that's what it's all about!**

**Why you have to remain open to acquiring new habits**

We have a final thought for you in this slice. It is likely that you will not acquire all of the good habits you need right at the start of your diet. Certainly we did not, because we kept discovering new ideas about weight loss, and hence habits we wanted to acquire – and we still keep discovering them after several years of maintenance. But the earlier new habits are established, the better. And it is particularly advantageous to establish them before you get to your target weight. Why? Because those new habits are going to make it much easier for you to get through the tricky time just after you have reached your target weight. And they will also make it much easier to maintain your weight. More about this later, when we focus on weight maintenance, especially in slice 29.

# Slice 3

# Get motivated and stay motivated

Motivation is at the heart of any attempt to lose weight and keep that weight off, so motivation is obviously important! It is no exaggeration to say that without motivation, your diet is probably doomed to failure – that's why this slice is early in our book.

The slice falls into four sections:
• What is motivation?
• Why does motivation matter so much at the start of your diet?
• How do you get motivated and stay motivated?
• How do you keep your motivation thriving when things go wrong?

Later in the book, we also have much to say about how motivation helps you stick at it when you have reached your target weight – when 'all' you have to do is stay at that weight for the rest of your life. That's in slice 30.

**What is motivation?**
Something 'motivates' you when it increases your desire to act in a certain way. Note that motivation is not the same as willpower. The difference is neatly summed up by the expression 'The spirit is willing, but the flesh is weak.' In other words, you have the desire to do something (you have the motivation), but you just can't make yourself do it (you don't have the willpower). Although motivation and willpower are not the same, the two are related, as we will see later in this slice.

**Why does motivation matter so much at the start of your diet?**
Willpower is the ability to control your mind and body so that you do something. If you want to lose weight, you will probably have to use your willpower to put a lot of effort into the goal of losing weight. You might imagine that having willpower is enough, but usually it is not. For nearly all of us, and in nearly all situations, we need a powerful *desire* to do something to 'fire up' our willpower and make it work well. That powerful desire is motivation, so motivation is of great importance to the dieter.

Motivation is particularly important at the start of your diet, simply to get your diet launched at a time when negative thoughts can go through your head. Negative thoughts could include:

'I'm cross with myself for getting overweight.'

'This is just my latest diet – I have done lots of diets in the past and have always put the weight back on.'

'I am out of control.'

That means that right at the start of your diet, you may have a problem. Motivation thrives on being positive, but you may have all of these negative thoughts kicking around in your head – thoughts that are *reducing* your motivation! Now is therefore clearly the time to look at how to get motivated.

**How do you get motivated and stay motivated?**

Much of this book is about non-magical solutions to real-world problems we have come across and about how to ease those problems by working things out in advance. The key to making these non-magical solutions work is willpower, and the key to firing up your willpower is to have motivation. So at the root of all this good stuff is a need to get motivated.

We think that one of the best writers about motivation for dieters is Judith Beck. We highly recommend her book *The Beck Diet Solution*, in which she suggests you make a long, detailed list of the benefits for you of losing weight. She says that the best time to write such a list of benefits is right at the start of your diet. Also, she recommends reading the list every morning, to keep the benefits to you of losing weight in the front of your mind.

Let's look at the idea of a list of benefits a little more with some chat time. It's a conversation we had a long time ago – before we even got to our target weights.

*CHAT TIME*

*STEVE: Could you give me some examples from your own list of benefits?*

*CAROLINE: Certainly. Bear in mind that lists of benefits should be long and detailed, but here are my two main benefits. The first is the serious one – to avoid getting diabetes. I am at high risk for a lot of reasons, but the only one I can do anything about is my weight. It isn't very motivating, though, because, apart from an annual check which tells me I still haven't got diabetes, there's nothing that is always in the front of my mind, motivating me.*

*STEVE: That's the serious one. Does that mean that the other is not a serious one?*

*CAROLINE: In a way, yes. Maybe it's better to describe it as more frivolous. Much more fun and motivating on a day-to-day level has been thinking that I want to be able to wear clothes I like – not just clothes that hide my bulges! The idea that I will be able to get rid of the 'fat clothes' and buy new and flattering ones is really motivating. A bit frivolous, I suppose!*

*STEVE: Frivolous maybe, but helpful at keeping motivation going for an awful lot of people.*

*CAROLINE: You're probably right. So what about you? What do you have on your list of benefits?*

*STEVE: I think the biggest benefit I see of losing weight is to be able to walk reasonably comfortably again. In the beginning, my knees were painful, and I had to walk with a stick. The physiotherapist told me that if I lost weight, the weight bearing down on my knees would reduce, so the pain would reduce, so I would be able to walk further and more comfortably. It's getting better, but there's still a long way to go.*

Being clear about the benefits of losing weight is a really useful tool, but it is not enough on its own. We have often met people in real life and on online forums for whom losing weight would clearly be beneficial, but they are still overweight, and they still ask how they can get motivated.

The simple answer is that motivation has to come from within us. That burning desire to *do* something that is going to fire up our willpower to actually lose weight must come from somewhere between our own ears! There are things you can do to encourage that burning desire – that motivation – to thrive. And best of all is to be positive, because **motivation thrives on positive thinking**.

**Your first positive and motivating thought** is that you must already be quite motivated because you have chosen to acquire a book about dieting. You have spent some of your precious, hard-earned cash on buying it, and now you are spending valuable time reading it. All of this is an excellent start (and, of course, an excellent choice of book!).

**Your second positive and motivating thought** is that you are not going to be making the biggest mistake that most dieters make. That biggest mistake is to think that you will get through this 'diet' quickly by eating a small amount until you get to the weight you want to be. Then, with a sigh of relief, you can go back to eating 'normally' – which means the way you ate before you started your diet. To the best of our knowledge, this rarely (if ever) works. If someone does get down to their target weight but then switches back to their pre-diet eating habits, they'll return to their pre-diet weight – how could it be otherwise? So, almost certainly, you are going to be disappointed if you approach your diet in that way; you will become yet another 'yo-yo dieter'. If you are not quite sure about this, just think – have you tried dieting like that before? Did it work? See what we mean?

That second positive thought may not have *looked* all that positive! But the good news is that having the knowledge that yo-yo dieting *cannot work* enables you to think positively about *what will work* this time. We want you to ask yourself some questions:
'Is this your first diet?'
'If you dieted before, did you lose the weight you wanted to?'
'However much you did lose before, did you keep that weight off?'
If the answer to any of those questions is 'no', then the next (more searching) questions are:
'Do you know what went wrong?'
'Why do you think it will be different this time if you do the same thing again?'

We have had to answer these questions ourselves, and we know that they are not easy questions to answer. But you have something valuable that we did not – you have this book, which will help you to discover the answers you need this time. This is all positive and motivating stuff – you are thinking about what is going to work for you, and you know that you have help in your hand. And, what's more, you know that that help was written by two people who have made the whole journey themselves – from decades of yo-yo dieting to eventual success.

Let's look at another example of positive thinking, with some more chat time.

*CHAT TIME*

*CAROLINE: Of course, you, Steve, are a prime example of someone who showed the power of positive thinking to boost motivation, and from the very start of your diet too.*

*STEVE: I am?*

*CAROLINE: Yes, you are.*

*STEVE: Well, in those days, before I met you to educate me, I knew next to nothing about positive thinking or motivation.*

*CAROLINE: Maybe you were born with both. But the fact remains that when you signed up to Nutracheck, you chose the username 'stevelosing60kilos' – not, for example, 'fatboysteve'. The username 'stevelosing60kilos' made it clear to you, and to everyone else, that you were in the business of losing weight and, what's more, you were going to lose a lot of weight (nearly ten stone).*

*STEVE: So you think that having that username made me see myself as someone who was in charge of his weight – not just as someone who wanted to lose weight?*

*CAROLINE: I'm sure of it. And being in charge of your own weight was an important part of your life that became motivating in itself – it motivated you to do all the things that fit with being in charge of your own weight. Being careful with portion sizes, for example.*

We said above that it was good to be positive because motivation loves positive thinking. The opposite is true too – it is bad to be negative because **motivation is weakened by negative thinking**.

People can say things that illustrate underlying negative thinking. For example, 'I don't like rabbit food' and 'Diet food is boring.' These phrases (and many others) may be said in a light-hearted way, and they may seem harmless enough. But using phrases like these quietly works on us, persuading us that eating certain foods is good or bad. In the case of 'rabbit food', we are being worked on to dislike salad ingredients; that is a pity, because the negativity is reducing our motivation to eat foods that are a useful, low-calorie part of our diet.

Another example of the problems of negative thinking is if thinking about your weight always makes you have the negative thought that you are a 'fat failure'. If you think like that, you may not be motivated to get on the scales at all. We believe this is not at all helpful, because it is much easier to lose weight if you weigh yourself regularly. On the other hand, if you are positive and see yourself as 'someone who is in charge of their own weight', it is only natural to want to know your weight. Seeing how your weight changes becomes a useful tool, which gives interesting and important information. You will then be motivated, and your willpower will be even more powerful.

If you think negatively, shifting your thoughts to the positive can be quite a job. But once you do it, you will be pleased with yourself, and you should give yourself praise and a pat on the back. And that's motivating too!

**How do you keep your motivation thriving when things go wrong?**
Nobody has ever dieted and lost weight in immaculate straight lines, from start weight to target weight, and then for the many years of maintenance. Things are sure to go wrong! Common ways that things go wrong are:

• We seem to be doing everything right, but our bodies 'misbehave' and do not deliver the weight loss we hoped they would. The usual reason for this is because our bodies are not machines. We take in a vast assortment of fuel, we use energy in a vast number of different ways, we carry our (heavy) waste products around with us, we get rid of those waste products at various times, and many women have physical changes every month or so. The complexity of all of this going on means our weight bobs up and down for no apparent reason or, most annoyingly of all, stays on a plateau for ages.

• As a diet continues, many people find that their motivation decreases. The excitement of initial fast weight loss gets less, and as that excitement gets less, so does motivation. Motivation often comes and goes for no apparent reason but, let's face it, where dieting is concerned, mostly we notice it going!

• Motivation seems to evaporate in the face of favourite foods, social occasions, and comfort eating.

These (and other) ways of going wrong can be demotivating, and if you start saying things to yourself such as 'I'm never going to lose this weight,' then that negative thinking will certainly not help your motivation. So just when you need your motivation to help get you through a difficult time, motivation ceases to fire up your willpower, and your willpower is no longer enough to overcome those negative thoughts. The risk is that you will get fed up and give up.

The burning question, therefore, is **how do you keep your motivation thriving when things go wrong?** Motivation is a personal thing, but here are some ideas that you may be able to work on to boost your own motivation.

**Go back to your list of benefits** (the list of benefits of losing weight, which we talked about earlier). The list is extremely helpful when things start to go wrong. Don't just read it, but really work with it. Perhaps write it out again in order of importance of the benefits or in order of the benefits that are most motivating for you right now. Perhaps group it into different categories, such as health, self-image, or what will be more fun when you've lost weight. It may also be a good time to review whether you want to add to (or subtract from) your list of benefits.

We have both found working with our lists of benefits to be an immediate injection of positivity and motivation. We both have a copy of *The Beck Diet Solution* on our bookshelves, and you could do much worse than get one yourself (and, no, we don't get a commission from Dr Beck – we just like the book!).

**Look at what you've achieved already.** Consider how much weight you have lost already. Whether it is a pound, a stone, or ten stone, it is progress in the right direction. It wasn't easy to lose it, and you don't want to undo your good work!

**Just for a moment, think negatively.** Suppose you stop dieting right now; what happens next? You put on the weight you so carefully and painstakingly shed. What next? You can't fit into the clothes you are wearing now. Then you'll either have to get out clothes you hoped you'd never wear again or buy clothes that are bigger. How heavy will you be when your weight gain stops? If moving around is problematic because of pain or your current size, how much worse will that get? What will your quality of life be like if you put the weight back on? What would you like your life to be like? And we're back to that list of benefits of losing weight again – we don't stay negative for long!

**Look forward to what you want to achieve.** Many people have an item or a style of clothing they would like to get back into or buy. Look at it and imagine yourself in it – isn't that worth forgoing that bar of chocolate for?!

**Change the way you think of motivation.** How you think of motivation will help you to harness it and increase it in the hard times.

It can be quite a problem if you think of your motivation in the same way as you think about time – you spend time doing something and that time is gone forever. If you see motivation in that way, and feel that your motivation is slipping, then things do indeed look hopeless. And it's tempting to think 'That's it, I just don't have what it takes to diet' and get fed up and give up. So try to look at motivation in other ways, such as:

• Think of your motivation to diet in the same way as a friendship – a friendship that anybody can build between themselves and their diet. You may fall out from time to time, but, with a little thought and effort, you can rebuild your friendship. Sometimes the relationship even emerges strengthened.

• Think of your motivation to diet in the same way as energy – everyone's energy levels fluctuate. Some things drain your energy, but there are other things you can do that *build up* your energy.

Both of the above ways of looking at motivation mean that you no longer have the negative thought that you are in the hopeless situation of your motivation being permanently lacking.

Those were some ideas on how to keep your motivation thriving; we hope that some or all of them will be useful. Specifically, we hope that the ideas will help you to see how, if your motivation to diet slips, you have a real choice. That choice is whether to let your diet just wither away or try to work out what went wrong and pick yourself up, wiser, more thoughtful, and freshly motivated.

This has been a long slice, but (trying not to be big-headed) we are specialists in this area, and we would strongly encourage you to read and re-read the slice until all of its messages have struck home. As we said a few pages ago, motivation is at the heart of any attempt to lose weight and keep that weight off, so we think this is an excellent slice to get to grips with. We suggest that, on your list of benefits, you write 're-read slice 3', so if your motivation needs a boost, you can come back here to get one!

# Slice 4

# Understand emotional eating

Emotional eating is a strange idea; why should our emotions affect how we eat? But for a lot of people that is exactly what happens – they want to eat because they are feeling sad, or lonely, or bored, or angry, or anxious, or overwhelmed. When we talk about this kind of emotional eating – eating in response to your mood at that moment – we are going to call it 'spur-of-the-moment' emotional eating.

But perhaps even more difficult to understand is the notion that there might be longstanding emotional reasons why people don't *want* to be slim – even though they *think* they want to lose weight. When we talk about this kind of emotional eating – where eating patterns or beliefs about yourself have been affecting you for a long time – we are going to call it 'longstanding' emotional eating.

Of course, people being people, it isn't always as simple as the above. For example, there may be people who sometimes eat in response to a spur-of-the-moment emotion – for longstanding reasons! Also, some people (Steve, for example) react to strong emotions by *losing* their appetite, but this is unusual, and we are not going to pursue it further.

Perhaps we should also say here that there is another emotional eating problem for the dieter, which is eating in response to social pressures. That one is so important that it has a slice of its own – slice 10.

We suspect that emotional eating of some kind plays a part in weight gain for many of us. This slice will therefore be key to successful weight loss for a large number of people. It will help you to understand the subject of emotional eating, and slice 20 will help you to do something about it. Even if you think emotional eating is not relevant to you, we would encourage you to read these emotional eating slices anyway. And we would especially encourage you to read these emotional eating slices if you are someone who has previously lost weight and then put it back on, and even more especially if you have done that over and over again. It is worth considering whether there is a longstanding eating pattern that has contributed to this 'yo-yo dieting'.

We are not considering in this book the true eating disorders, such as anorexia nervosa and bulimia. Suffice it to say that if you are vomiting or purging as a weight control mechanism, or if you feel your eating is otherwise out of control, this is dangerous for your health and it would be best to discuss it with your GP or mental health worker.

## Spur-of-the-moment emotional eating

If you are spur-of-the-moment emotionally eating, then somewhere along the line, you have confused emotions with hunger and have got into the habit of eating (or drinking) in order to feel better. The emotions that trigger eating are different for all of us. It is very helpful to think about what they are for you because then you can begin to do something about it.

If you are an emotional eater, you are likely to have noticed that you rarely turn to spinach salad in moments of distress! Far more likely is that your emotional eating concentrates on highly processed carbohydrates – mainly sweet and fatty items. These foods will probably give you some immediate relief because they fire off the 'this is nice' centres in your brain, which damps down the 'I feel bad' messages for a bit, and that feels good. This teaches you that eating can damp down the unpleasant emotions.

The more often you eat to make yourself feel better, the less you experience the fact that painful feelings are not actually dangerous – like hunger itself, those painful feelings will come and go. This means that next time that you are unhappy, you are more likely to think that you must eat in order to feel better.

If you are not sure whether you emotionally overeat or not, it might help to ask yourself some questions:
• Last time I overate, was I content, involved in what I was doing, or with pleasant people? That sounds as if it wasn't emotional eating.
• Last time I overate, was I bored, lonely, sad, angry, frustrated, scared, or any combination of them? That sounds like emotional overeating. If this doesn't help you to know whether it was emotional eating, you could put it the other way round:
• Last time I was bored, lonely, sad, angry, frustrated, or scared, was I also hungry or eating? Again, that points towards emotional overeating.

Spur-of-the-moment emotional eating is common. It slows dieting down or, worse, means people give up. In slice 20, we will look in more detail at ways of handling (and minimising) your emotional eating once you have identified it.

## Longstanding emotional eating

The simplest kind of longstanding emotional eating happens because of patterns of eating that have been part of your life for so long that you cannot imagine changing them. In fact, if you think that you shouldn't even be asked to change these eating patterns, that is a big clue that there is an emotional element to it!

A typical example is that you 'must finish everything on your plate'. If you automatically scrape your plate clean because your mother told you to, or if she was pleased with you when you did, then it's less likely that you have learned to spontaneously stop eating when you have had enough. Unless you consciously change this habit, it is likely to sabotage your efforts to lose weight time and time again.

A common anxiety is that if you become thinner, you will lose that 'safe' feeling that some people have when they are overweight. You may believe you will become more likely to be the subject of unwanted (or dangerous) sexual attention, for example. If you consider that your overeating and weight gain is due to reasons like this, you may be able to work through it on your own – simply recognising it is the first step to changing it. In slice 20 there are some ideas to help you think about this some more.

**Congratulations!** If you are still reading, you have probably already taken the first step in solving your emotional eating problem. You have understood that sometimes you eat for emotional reasons and that this is not going to help you lose weight and keep it off. This not-so-simple step of understanding what is happening is vital because without it, you will probably never find ways to overcome your emotional eating.

The second step is also vital and equally tricky. It is to understand a pretty stark message, where there is no way to make it fun or amusing. You have a choice to make. The emotions and experiences driving you to eat may be very strong, very sad, and very deep. All emotions are valid and are there because you feel them. Your choice, however, is either (1) to use them as an excuse not to lose weight or (2) to find a way to tackle them because you want (and deserve) to be a healthy weight. If only there was another way. If only there could be a get-out-of-jail-free card for people who have had it tough and learned the long and difficult lesson that food temporarily comforts and soothes when nothing else does. But sadly there is no other way, and there is no get-out-of-jail-free card.

The trouble is that your body doesn't know or care *why* you are eating. It merely adds the calories as they mount up. It doesn't make any difference to your body whether you are comfort eating because your father never loved you or because you just broke a fingernail or because you had a bad day at work. To your body, it's all just calories. And as we want to help you lose weight and keep it off, we can't pretend otherwise. That's the really tough bit: if you are eating emotionally, it will get in the way of weight loss and the long-term maintenance of that weight loss. Your choice is to use emotional eating as an excuse to eat more or to find a way to manage it. We hope that you are going to choose the latter.

There will then be further emotional issues to get to grips with once you move into maintenance of your weight loss. We will discuss these in slice 31.

# Slice 5

# Understand self-defeating thoughts

Losing weight is not easy. It is hard enough to change what you eat and re-organise your life, sometimes without much support from your friends and family. So the last thing you want is to be defeated by the person who is nearest to you – yourself!

What are we talking about? How can you be defeated by *yourself*? Well, dieters are defeated by themselves if they have a thought that stops them from getting on with their diet in the way they want to. Here is a simple example – if you constantly think 'I have always been fat, and I know that I always *will be* fat,' then you will probably find it difficult to start and continue with a diet – you have defeated yourself.

Self-defeating thoughts come when we are feeling less motivated, and they can be hard to recognise. They can be at least partly true – for example, 'I've never done a diet that's succeeded before' may well have some truth in it. We can also fool ourselves into believing that a thought that is really an opinion is actually a fact. So if your complete thought was 'I've never done a diet that's succeeded before, so this one won't either,' you may have a toxic combination of something that could be true with a belief that what is only an (unkind) opinion is actually an (unhelpful) fact.

What self-defeating thoughts have in common is that they can push you off course and stop you getting to your target weight – and that is an extremely important goal to you (you know that because you are reading this book!).

**Identifying self-defeating thoughts**
A self-defeating thought is the kind of thing someone critical of you might actually say – using the example above, 'You've always been fat.' Look out for those thoughts and see them for what they are! A thought is likely to be self-defeating if
• it makes you feel bad, or
• it gives you a reason/excuse to give up on your diet, or
• it's something you'd never say to your best friend if she was trying to lose weight, or
• it says something critical or unpleasant about you.

Please do not underestimate the power of these self-defeating thoughts. They come from the person who knows you best of all (you) and from the person who knows where you are weakest (that's you again!). Self-defeating thoughts come to us all at some point, and some people get them more than others. Having identified a self-defeating thought, the trick is to learn to deal with it, and that is what the rest of this slice is about.

**Countering self-defeating thoughts**
Let's look at another example of a self-defeating thought. Say that you want to lose some weight, but you think, 'I went out on Friday night and ate and drank far too much. I am a failure. Clearly I will never lose weight, so I might as well give up.' This is a common thought but not a helpful one because, obviously, it does not lead to weight loss! Here are five steps to a more helpful approach in this situation:
1. **Motivate yourself.** Remind yourself why you want to lose weight in the first place.
2. **Recognise that this is a self-defeating thought.** Recognise that your thought is making you feel bad, but it is simply a thought – a self-defeating thought. It is not a fact that you need to act on.
3. **Understand why the self-defeating thought does not help you to achieve your goal.** Tell yourself that giving up is *definitely* not going to help you lose weight.
4. **Find a countering (helpful) thought in place of the self-defeating thought.** Ask yourself, 'If I had a friend who particularly wanted to lose weight and she was telling me those thoughts about overdoing things, being a failure, and giving up, *what would I say to her now*?' Perhaps it might be 'One evening of overeating does not ruin your diet, but giving up because of it certainly would!'
5. **Decide what to do next.** Decide what you need to do to help you reach your weight loss goal. Maybe this could be to make a plan to stay within calories just for today.

These steps would be helpful in this particular situation and also helpful when you find yourself thinking, for any reason, 'I might as well give up.' In fact, using these steps is also a general approach that you can take to deal with any self-defeating thought.

Everyone will have self-defeating thoughts that are specific to them and their situation. But there is one self-defeating thought that is so common and so potentially damaging that we are going to give it a section of its own.

### 'It's not fair'

There are many aspects of dieting that seem not to be fair! Examples of what can feel 'not fair' are (1) having a sweet tooth, (2) not being able to stop at one biscuit, (3) having a strong preference for fatty foods, and (4) not being able to tolerate the feeling of being hungry. And it's true that if you don't have a sweet tooth, can stop at just one small portion of a high-calorie food, don't like chips, pastry, or Indian takeaways, and don't mind feeling hungry for a bit – then losing weight is going to be much easier for you. Let's be honest here – if you are a fortunate person like that, you are unlikely to be reading this book!

Things that don't seem fair can also be true, but that probably doesn't make you feel any better. After all, it may be true that you don't have the spare calories to go on an all-inclusive cruise for your fortieth birthday, but it still feels unfair. Even if you know something is true, you can easily start to think that it's not fair, that you are being unjustly punished, and that you are just going to go ahead and do what you wanted to do anyway!

What you just ended up with was a self-defeating thought. We said earlier that recognising self-defeating thoughts can be tricky, but recognising them does get easier as you get the hang of doing it. And a top tip is that any thought that is about both fairness and dieting is likely to be a self-defeating one!

Let's look at another example of how to use our five steps to overcome a self-defeating thought. The thought this time came from Sue, and it's an 'it's not fair' sort of thought. She said that her partner Paul had a bigger calorie allowance than she did, and he could eat whatever he liked and not put on weight.

We think this is a useful example because it is absolutely true that there is usually quite a difference between the calorie allowances of men and women. But it can still be a sore point for a woman if her male partner sits there every night eating a lot of snacks that are so calorific that *she* just cannot squeeze them into her diet planning. It's no wonder that women can think that it's not fair. So here are the same five steps, which Sue can apply to this thought:

1. **Motivate yourself.** We suggest the same powerful motivator as before – Sue could remind herself why she wants to lose weight.

2. **Recognise that this is a self-defeating thought.** Again, this is similar to what we said before. Sue can reflect that, irritating though it may be to think that Paul seems to be able to eat what he likes, it is just a thought. She does not need to act on it.

**3. Understand why the self-defeating thought does not help you to achieve your goal.** Sue can try to see that dwelling on the 'unfairness' is not going to help her to keep to her diet. She can think, 'If I eat the same amount as Paul, I won't reach my goal and – worse – I will put weight back on.'

**4. Find a countering (helpful) thought in place of the self-defeating thought.** Caroline admits to using the following countering thought about Steve: 'So what if Steve can eat and drink more than me and still lose weight? The person who matters is *me*! I have to stay within my calorie allowance if I want to lose weight.' Sue could use the same thought (of course about Paul, not Steve!). Also, there is no particular reason to use just one countering thought. Whenever 'fairness' threatens to lead you off track, another useful thought can be, 'I have freely chosen to lose weight for lots of good reasons. Fairness is not the point – keeping my eye on the goal is the point.'

**5. Decide what to do next.** This will depend on Sue's own situation. Perhaps she could decide to plan meals more carefully, so they are enjoyable and filling but still within calories.

If you are ever tempted to see something about your diet as 'not fair', we suggest that you have a go at understanding the situation better by using this five-step approach. Every time you use this approach, it will get quicker. In the end, it will just seem like 'common sense', and you may come to see (at least some) self-defeating thoughts as no more than excuses.

**Sharing your self-defeating thoughts**
We have one last thought in this slice. It's all too easy, especially in a world of social media, to share our self-defeating thoughts. Pretty soon these thoughts may have been shared with a lot of people – family, friends, and people we scarcely know on online forums. The problem can be that if you share a thought often enough, especially with people who want to be supportive, then that thought begins to feel completely normal and not something that you need to deal with. Generally, therefore – and we know this might be difficult – we think that it is best to work on your own at countering your self-defeating thoughts, while sharing them as little as possible.

# Slice 6

# Decide on your approach to weight loss

This title sounds nice, but what does it actually mean? An example of an 'approach to weight loss' is whether you are going to (1) try to lose a lot of weight quickly or (2) try to lose weight slowly and gradually. You can take different approaches to the speed of weight loss, and the approach you take will influence your life for a long time and may even decide whether your weight loss succeeds or fails. And that's just one example.

What we are going to do in this slice is look at different approaches that you can take and give you some guidance on how you could decide. The slice is early in the book to highlight what you need to be thinking about in following your diet. It may be even more important for those people, like us, with a history of trying to lose weight and failing. This time you may want to do things differently.

Just to be clear: this slice flags up some big issues to think about before you start your diet. All of the detail within these issues and what you can actually *do* to help your weight loss to succeed are covered in part 2 of the book.

**What priority are you prepared to give to weight loss in your life?**
You've probably already discovered that losing weight is difficult – that may be why you are reading a book about it. We said earlier that losing weight is often compared to the difficulty of giving up smoking, but for many, it's even worse than that. At least with smoking it's possible (even if difficult) to give up entirely. But you can't give up food entirely!

Because weight loss is difficult, we found that it was important to make losing weight a high priority in our own lives. We knew from experience that when we didn't do that, we didn't lose weight (or, worse, we put it back on). Certainly, when we started on what we hoped were our final diets, we realised that weight loss would not 'just happen' because we wanted it to. We therefore gave weight loss a high priority, and we continue to do so in maintenance. If you don't think you can do that, perhaps you might look back at slice 3 to try to boost your motivation.

However – before you start to think that we mean you can never again have a meal that is high-calorie, never again have a piece of birthday cake, or have to give up crisps forever – no, that is not what we mean! Caroline has regular social events that include big meals, and Steve's work means he is away from home and has little choice about what he is served for several days a month. On these occasions, both of us enjoy eating food that we no longer eat often. Giving dieting a high priority doesn't mean *never* having high-calorie foods – but it does mean being careful. It means (1) having high-calorie foods rarely enough to avoid starting to put on weight or (2) cutting back on what we eat before (or after) a big meal to compensate for it. Such examples of being careful are what we describe as exercising 'constant vigilance', and you will hear this phrase a lot more as you read the book!

## How many other big changes do you intend to make during your weight-loss journey?

A common approach to weight loss is to see it as an opportunity to improve general health. This might involve *reducing* intake of salt, sugar, biscuits, alcohol, saturated fat, caffeine, etc.; *increasing* intake of unprocessed food, fibre, 'good fats', brown rice, micronutrients, etc.; *increasing* exercise; and even *giving up* smoking.

The difficulty with trying to make a lot of changes at the same time is that life becomes complicated. There is so much to think about, to buy, and to monitor that it is easy to lose sight of the main objective, which is to lose weight. Some people can manage to do everything, but many can't – and those are the people who can end up making various beneficial changes to their lives but failing to actually lose any weight.

In our own cases, we kept in mind that by far the most important thing while dieting was to focus on the calories. Steve's motto was 'Keep It Simple', and he concentrated on calorie reduction almost exclusively. Caroline also concentrated on calories, but she also made sure she had a well-balanced and nutritious diet within her calorie allowance.

To a large extent, focusing on calories leads anyway to a 'healthy diet'. The 'unhealthy' foods (such as biscuits, cakes, alcohol, and saturated fats) tend to be higher in calories and the 'healthy' foods (vegetables, salad, lean meats, pulses, and fruit) tend to be lower in calories.

Thinking about how complicated you can make your dieting is important. Only *you* know whether you can achieve several (difficult) things in your life at the same time. It comes down to what priority you are prepared to give to weight loss – can you really give it a high priority and *also* give a high priority to other goals in your life? *You* may be able to, but we certainly didn't think that *we* could.

**What sort of diet will you follow?**
You have a vast choice. We are not going to name diets here because many diets become popular, then fade into obscurity when they are overtaken by something else. Anything we mention by name will probably be laughably dated a year after the book is published. Well, OK, we'll just name one: does anyone remember the Cabbage Soup Diet?

When deciding which diet to follow, we would strongly suggest that you keep in mind something we think is one of the most important points in the whole book: **a diet can only work if it restricts your calories**. If it is not clear that a diet is based on eating fewer calories than you are burning, then you should be cautious about following it.

There are, however, many diets that do not include the counting of calories. Instead, they might specify foods that must not be eaten or foods that can be eaten only at certain times or diets that measure 'points' rather than calories. Some of these diets are well-established and popular. But if you lose weight on them, it can *only be* because they are helping you to restrict your calories, so you are consuming fewer calories than you are burning. This is simple biology, not an amazing miracle diet! We will look at these diets in more detail in slice 8, but we just wanted to mention them here.

We would also suggest that you don't get too excited about any particular new diet. It may have the support of a 'celebrity', there may be a long line of 'eminent doctors' swearing that it is 'scientifically proven', but a diet is never as amazingly successful as the publicity says it will be. If it was so successful, there would no more obesity in the world (whatever date you are reading this – is there still obesity in the world? Mmmm, we thought there would be!). In the dieting business it doesn't do any harm to be a little cynical.

Diets that might work fall into three types:
• diets where you eat less,
• diets where you eat different foods, and
• diets where you eat less and eat different foods.
You can add exercise to any of them.

Diets – of any of those types – can work, as long as you are eating fewer calories than you are burning (see above). But the trick is to find the one that can work *for you*. Dieting is a personal matter, and what works for one person may not work for somebody else. You might hate being hungry, so diets involving severe calorie reduction, including spells of fasting, probably won't be for you. You might be physically disabled, so diets involving a lot of exercise might not be possible for you. You might dislike counting calories, so calorie-counting systems are out. And so on and so on.

To use ourselves as examples, we are quite different people in many ways. But what we do have in common is a love of cooking, a liking of all sorts of food and drink, a dislike of vigorous exercise, an enthusiasm for numbers, a deep-seated belief in science, and a reluctance to attend regular diet group meetings. So it was only natural that we both ended up on diets that involved exploring all sorts of cooking with low-calorie ingredients, strict calorie counting, modest walking for exercise, and careful recording. We both used an online service (*Nutracheck*) to help with the counting and recording, and that's how we met, on their message board. The diet we used was successful because it suited our personal preferences.

Something else that we are fond of saying is **the best diet for you is the one that you will stick to!** This may seem obvious, but no diet can work if you can only do it for a couple of weeks – it has to be something that suits you, so you will be happy to follow it for a long time.

Finally, despite thinking hard about which is the diet for you, do be prepared to find that the diet you have selected turns out not to suit you very well after all. It may be OK at first, but then your enthusiasm wanes, your weight loss stalls, and you know that you are not going to be able to rekindle your interest in the diet. In that case, don't flog a dead horse – try something else. You might even want to identify two diets right at the start, so you know that you have a Plan B that you can switch to quite quickly.

### How quickly do you intend to lose weight?
That might sound like a daft question! The obvious answer might be 'as quickly as possible!' And that answer may be even more obvious if you have chosen a 'miracle diet' – because that will almost certainly come with a promise of fast and easy weight loss. There are, however, two big problems with losing weight quickly.

**It is likely (not certain, but likely) to mean that any weight you do lose will be quickly regained.** For what it is worth, we have never yet heard of anybody who lost a lot of weight quickly and then kept it off for a long time. And that is not surprising, given what we said in slices 2 and 3 about why quick weight *loss* is usually followed by quick weight *gain*. If you don't quite remember the reasons, it might be a good idea to turn back and refresh your memory.

**Losing weight quickly is difficult.** Why? When we lose weight, what we are doing is consuming less fuel than our body needs, and that is called a calorie deficit. To lose a pound of fat, we need a calorie deficit of about 3,500 calories. So if we intend to lose a pound in a week, we will need a calorie deficit of about 500 calories a day. If we intend to lose *two pounds* in a week, we are going to need a calorie deficit of 1,000 calories a day. That is a massive reduction for most people!

A calorie deficit of 1,000 calories a day is particularly drastic for most women, because their bodies often need only 1,500 to 2,000 calories a day, so they are depriving themselves of a large part of what their bodies need. Bodies usually fight back, and you can become tired, hungry, and lacking in proper nourishment. And that is to lose two pounds a week. Many people attempt to lose three, four, or more pounds a week, and that can be the best part of impossible, involving eating very little and *also* burning off calories by intensive exercise. They do not stick to diets like that for very long!

We did say earlier that the best diet for you is the one that suits your own preferences and that you will stick to. And we still think that's true and, of course, the choice is entirely yours. But we do believe that, whatever your preferences, you have a choice between:

• Losing weight quickly (if you can) and then, having reached your target weight, having to think afresh about how you are going to maintain. This will be a particularly big change if you have followed a 'powders and potions' sort of diet.

• Losing weight more slowly, tweaking what you eat as you continue to lose more weight, so your diet will be more sustainable in the long term. Having reached your target weight, you can merely tweak your diet a little more as you move into maintenance. Slower weight loss will also give you more time to acquire useful new habits for the long term.

We think that losing a pound a week is perfectly reasonable. If you are following a doable weight-reduction diet, so you are happy to follow it week after week, then in a year of one-pound-a-week losses you will have lost getting on for four stone. If you want to be particularly ambitious and you are unusually motivated, then two pounds a week is still the most you should attempt to lose. If you manage to follow that for a year, that will give you a huge loss of seven and a half stone.

That sort of loss will satisfy almost everyone. If you are thinking of attempting to lose weight more quickly, we do suggest that you discuss it with your doctor before starting.

**Do you intend to put a lot of focus on exercise?**
The extremes here are (1) to intend to do a lot of exercise because you want it to be your most important weight-loss tool or (2) to intend not to do any exercise at all. The approach you adopt between these extremes will depend to some extent on your physical abilities and whether or not you like exercise.

If you are ready, willing, and able to do a lot of exercise, that's great. But although exercise is very useful as a calorie burner, it does have its limits. It takes a great deal of exercise to burn off a calorific meal, and so it is highly unlikely that you will be able to lose significant weight through exercise alone. We look at this in detail in slice 9, but the main message is that however keen you are on exercise, you will also almost certainly need to get interested in limiting the calories you consume.

On the other hand, if you don't want to (or can't) do any exercise, your weight loss will still happen, although it may be slower. Slice 23 covers how to increase your calories burned, and it will help you. We would also suggest that you continue to remain open to the possibility of doing at least some exercise, because your ability to do it (and your liking of it) may increase as your weight decreases. As examples, Caroline used to do no exercise to speak of and referred to herself as a 'sloth', and Steve could barely walk at all because of complications associated with his high body weight. A few years later, we were both at target weight, averaged 10,000 steps a day, and were fond of walks in the country. It's hardly pumping iron in a gym, but that walking was a valuable and pleasurable part of our weight control. It has also become a part of our general lifestyle change.

**How much planning do you intend to do?**
Planning particularly refers to shopping and cooking. Some people are spontaneous – they go round the supermarket and pick up what they fancy for the evening's meal. Other people figure out what they will be eating for the day ahead (or even for the week ahead).

The consensus (if there is a consensus in the world of dieting!) is that the more spontaneous approach makes dieting success less likely. The risk is that what you fancy on the spur of the moment will tend to be more calorific – few people will suddenly spot a head of celery in the supermarket and get an overwhelming urge to put it in their trolley. Even if you are counting calories as you go along, you may well find that you have eaten so many earlier in the day that what you eat later in the day pushes you into territory where you will gain weight, not lose it.

Our advice, in common with the advice of a lot of other people, is to plan your diet as much as you can (and we go into detail about this in slice 15). But then we would give that advice because we are much more planning personality types than spontaneous types.

If you do live your life spontaneously, it's probably not something you can switch on and off. But what we would suggest is, as much as possible, to plan *the food consumption part of your life* but stay spontaneous about your exercise. It can never be wrong to burst into an unexpected bout of calorie burning!

### Are you going to enlist the help of others with your diet?

Are you going to approach your diet by doing it all on your own, not telling anyone about it, maybe until they notice that you have lost a few pounds? Or are you going to tell everyone you know right from the beginning?

There are pros and cons to each. If you tell everybody and your diet fails almost as soon as you start, you may feel a little foolish (depending on what your friends and relatives are like) and possibly less keen to try again. But if you keep it to yourself, you will have nobody to help you if things start to go wrong. It depends on your own personality and the personalities of those around you. All we can offer as advice is to consider the enormous help that it can be, having someone in your corner – we talk about this in slice 11.

We would also suggest that you think about how your diet is going to affect your family. Are they all suddenly going to be eating what you are eating? Are they going to be supportive if you want to start going out for a walk every day? You are going to have a change of lifestyle here – what will your family's attitude be to that? We suggest that you talk to them before your diet even starts – the time to start talking is not when they are already fed up with what you are doing!

### How are you going to measure your progress?

We cover this elsewhere in the book (for example, in slice 24), but we wanted to highlight it here, before your diet even starts. We have said that dieting is difficult, and it is especially so without some regular welcome feedback that the diet is working. For many people, including ourselves, it's obvious how to get that regular welcome feedback – you hop onto the scales regularly (typically every week). If it's lower than the previous week, the diet is working!

But there are other ways of measuring progress, such as checking your waist measurement, noting your dress size, seeing whether a favourite item of clothing is fitting comfortably yet (taking photos of yourself can help with this), measuring your body fat percentage, or simply noticing how you feel.

Someone's preferred way of measuring depends, at least partly, on whether or not they are a 'numbers person'. We do suggest, however, that you would benefit from *some way* of measuring your progress. And also that whatever you are going to use to measure progress, you have a think about it now, ready for that important measurement at the very start of your diet. You will be referring back to that measurement for quite some time to come!

And finally, although we recognise that some people do have some success with non-weight measurements, for us to try to cover all such ways of measuring progress in this book would make the book unwieldy and hard to follow. We therefore make the assumption in our book that you will be measuring your progress in terms of body weight.

# Slice 7

# Decide on your target weight

We have already said that, although there are other ways of approaching it, this book is based on the idea of measuring diet progress by measuring weight. To do that, you need to know what your target weight is.

Your target weight is going to depend a lot on how tall you are. It's pretty obvious that somebody who is 6'3" will expect to weigh more than somebody who is 4'10". There is a well-known measurement that takes into account your height, and that's the body mass index (BMI). The BMI is widely used when doctors are assessing if your weight is acceptable.

There are plenty of online calculators that will work out your BMI for you. But you might be itching to know how to work out your BMI for yourself. If so, have a look at the chat time below. But if you're allergic to mathematics, just skip the chat and read on.

*CHAT TIME*

*CAROLINE: To find your BMI, take your weight and divide it by the square of your height. Just remember that your weight has to be in kilograms and your height has to be in metres.*

*STEVE: Although, if you search around the internet a bit, you should also be able to find online calculators in stones and pounds and feet and inches as well.*

*CAROLINE: But however you get your BMI, the next question is basically 'so what?'*

*STEVE: The usual table on that subject is:*
*BMI below 18.5: underweight*
*18.5 to 24.9: healthy weight (the NHS says 'ideal weight')*
*25 to 29.9: overweight*
*30 to 39.9: obese*
*40 and above: morbidly obese (in other words, very obese)*

*CAROLINE: It's true that BMI is far from perfect – for example, it can't show whether the weight you are carrying is muscle or bone or simply excess fat. But, for many people, the BMI is a good general guide.*

A good way of deciding on your target weight is simply to aim for a BMI in the 'ideal' band (18.5–24.9). You can then use one of those online calculators to tell you what weight you need to be to achieve that BMI. To use ourselves as examples, Caroline started with a BMI of 30 and set herself a target of a BMI of 25 (giving her a target weight of 10 st 6 lb), and Steve started with a BMI of 43 and also set a target of a BMI of 25 (giving him a target of 13 st 3 lb).

For us, those targets seemed reasonable. And once we got to our target weights, we realised that at those BMIs we did, indeed, look right and feel right. We had the added bonus that because doctors use BMI to assess whether body weight is OK, they stopped nagging us about our weight!

By now you might be thinking that this emphasis on setting a weight target based on your BMI is all a bit of a pain. But we both firmly believe that it is good to have a clear target and one that you can keep measuring yourself against as you lose weight. We think that having a measurable target is important – if your target is rather vague, such as 'I just want to feel better,' then it is easy to lose your focus. Losing weight can be tough, and in one of those tougher moments you may well say to yourself something like, 'Oh well, I do feel a bit better, so I think I'll stop now.' Nothing keeps you on track so much as having a clear target to go for – a number rather than something that is hard (or impossible) to measure.

**Making your weight-loss target less overwhelming**
It is often a good idea, especially if you have a lot of weight to lose, to set yourself a smaller weight-loss target. Then, when you have hit that one, you can set yourself another mini-target, and so on. Steve had some chat time about this with Robert, a friend of ours.

*CHAT TIME*

ROBERT: *I've never been a successful dieter! I have a lot to lose, so I set my target in the healthy BMI range.*

STEVE: *That sounds like a good approach.*

ROBERT: *I suppose it is. But I start my diet, and then as soon as anything goes wrong (like not losing any weight in a particular week), I look at the weight-loss mountain I have to climb. Then I think that if I have failed already, I have got no chance of reaching my target.*

*STEVE: Caroline and I call that the point when you get 'fed up and give up'.*

*ROBERT: Yes, that describes it nicely. But what can I do about it?*

*STEVE: We know many people who set small mini-targets, so they are not overwhelming. The first target is then easier to achieve, and you get a sense of achievement.*

*ROBERT: Oh, I see. And with that sense of achievement, it makes it easier to continue.*

*STEVE: That's the idea.*

*ROBERT: How much should these mini-targets be?*

*STEVE: Like with so many other aspects of dieting, it's a personal thing. Caroline and I both used this mini-target approach. Caroline set herself five-pound mini-targets and I set myself ten-pound mini-targets.*

*ROBERT: Didn't you get impatient, just losing in ten-pound chunks?*

*STEVE: I suppose that is a danger of setting mini-targets, but I don't think either of us got particularly impatient. I think we found regularly hitting our targets was nicely encouraging.*

*ROBERT: OK, sold! I'll give mini-targets a try.*

Splitting up your target weight loss into smaller amounts is a useful technique. It works for many people because it involves changing how you think. And changing how you think about things is an important part of dieting success. There are many more examples of that in this book.

We'll finish this slice with a single paragraph about an extraordinarily complex subject. To put it simply, it is important to set yourself a *realistic* target weight. If your target is very low (corresponding to an 'underweight BMI' of below 18.5), you may well find it extremely difficult to achieve that weight. More importantly, unless you are under medical supervision it is not usually safe to aim for such a target weight. This book is aimed at people who wish to keep their weight within a healthy range (broadly speaking that means a BMI of 18.5–24.9).

# Slice 8

# Understand the benefits of counting and recording calories

It may have already become clear as you read our book that we are big fans of calorie counting as a tool for sustainable weight loss. But why? Caroline had a chat with her friend Theresa on this subject, and here is an edited version of their discussion.

*CHAT TIME*

*THERESA: You do talk a lot about calorie counting and recording. Why do you like it so much?*

*CAROLINE: Perhaps the biggest reason is that it has worked so well for Steve and myself! We calorie counted our way down to our current healthy weights and have continued to calorie count our way through several years of maintaining our weight losses.*

*THERESA: But there are lots of other ways of losing weight, aren't there?*

*CAROLINE: Yes, there are, and many of them can work. But we think that calorie counting gives most people the best chance of success.*

*THERESA: Why is that?*

*CAROLINE: Let me start by asking you a question: what were the tricky bits about your previous diets? You must have had some – because I know that you have dieted several times before.*

*THERESA: How true! Well, the worst part was that I was deprived of what I really liked and I always had to eat the same low-calorie foods – it was boring.*

*CAROLINE: But did you just keep going, although it was a bit boring?*

*THERESA: No, I'm afraid not. It wasn't very long before I hit a patch where I didn't lose much weight, then I just got fed up and things sort of drifted.*

*CAROLINE: Hmmm, yes. And apart from being deprived and bored, was there anything else that was tricky with your previous diets?*

*THERESA: Yes. It made eating out a nightmare, whether it was in restaurants or other people's houses. Also, my life is different every day, so it was hard to eat in the same way every day. Basically, it was too inflexible.*

*CAROLINE: I'm glad we chose you for this chat time! You've neatly illustrated what scuppers dieting for most people. It's a combination of*
*1. feeling deprived and bored with what you are eating, and*
*2. not being able to be flexible about what you eat.*

[It's worth saying at this stage that there is something else that often scuppers diets, and that is not knowing what to do when weight loss slows down or even stops. But we will get to that later – in slice 25.]

*THERESA: OK, but why does calorie counting stop what you just mentioned from scuppering diets?*

*CAROLINE: To put it simply, if you do calorie counting and recording, and you do it in the right way, there is no need to feel deprived, no need to be bored with what you eat, and nothing stopping you from being on a diet and having a normal life.*

*THERESA: This is just too good to be true. You'll need to convince me about that!*

*CAROLINE: Right, here we go. The system we followed, and the one we recommend, is that you give yourself an allowance of calories you can eat every day. Then you simply count your calories throughout the day and make sure that you don't go over the allowance.*

THERESA: Is that it?

CAROLINE: Yes, that's it. It is a simple but powerful system.

THERESA: I can certainly see that it's simple, but how does it stop those two diet scupperers you mentioned?

CAROLINE: OK, first let's look at 'feeling deprived and bored with what you are eating'. Counting calories puts you in charge of what you 'spend' your allowance of calories on, so you can have what you really like, as long as it is counted as part of your total.

THERESA: Now that is too good to be true! You mean that if all I ate was crisps and chocolate but I stayed within my calorie allowance, I would still lose weight?!

CAROLINE. Yes. However, perhaps surprisingly, you would find that difficult to do, because crisps and chocolate aren't very sustaining. You would get hungry, possibly have sugar cravings, and be more than likely to eat something else as well. And it is the 'something else as well' that would take you over your calorie allowance. Even if you did manage, for a long time, to keep to your allowance by eating crisps and chocolate, you'd also become unwell – because it is a diet lacking in an awful lot of essential nutrients. So yes, you would lose weight if you could do it, although we have never heard of anybody who has actually managed it!

THERESA: Is this going in that diet book you're writing? I've never seen another diet book say anything like that!

CAROLINE: That's because our diet book is the best there is! But seriously, although the crisps and chocolate diet is bonkers, counting calories means that you don't have to give up your favourite foods. And also, because you can eat whatever you want (as long as it is within your calorie allowance), you can eat a much wider variety of food, and that stops you getting bored.

THERESA: That all sounds reasonable. And I imagine that when you count calories, you start to learn which foods have a *lot of calories for a small portion, so you have to be careful with them. Foods like butter, maybe?*

*CAROLINE: Absolutely right! And, on the other hand, you get good at knowing which foods have very few calories but give you a nice pile of food, so you can keep hunger away. While we're on a roll, let's look at the other diet scupperer: not being able to be flexible about what you eat. You have the—*

*THERESA: No, no, let me! I suppose if I am eating out somewhere and I know it's calorific, I can reduce calories in other meals I have that day?*

*CAROLINE: Yes, you can. And even if you are eating more away from home, you can have fewer calories on days when you are at home to compensate. So counting calories can help enormously in losing weight and in carrying on with your normal life.*

*THERESA: Thanks. That's really interesting and really useful. But there is one last point – I get that counting is useful, but why do I have to record it all? Is writing it down really going to help?*

*CAROLINE: Yes, it is going to help. There is research that backs that up – it seems that recording what you are eating and the calories in it tends to make you think more about what you are eating, to keep you 'honest' and to stop you misremembering what you have consumed. All of these help you to lose weight. It certainly worked that way for Steve and myself and for many other dieters we know.*

We hope that our chat time about calorie counting was useful. There were two things that Caroline and Theresa talked about that we would now like to explore further.

### Is it really so easy to count calories?
Although, in the chat, Caroline and Theresa both used the word 'simple' about counting calories, it is not always seen that way – people can be put off counting calories because of what they believe is the complexity and bother of doing it. But that thinking is largely outdated. Certainly, counting calories used to involve mechanical kitchen scales, books to

look up calories, and doing calculations by hand – and that was a big task. But nowadays, with electronic scales and lots of apps to do the hard work for you, it is not complicated, and it does not need any great ability in arithmetic.

## Other dieting systems can work

Near the start of the chat time, Theresa asked about other ways of losing weight. There *are* other ways, and many of them *can* work. So, in that case, if they can work, and especially if they seem to be even simpler than calorie counting, why bother with calorie counting?

The answer to this is in the phrase 'many of them *can* work'. There is no getting around the fact of biology that *the only way a diet can work* is if it is helping you to restrict your calories, so you are consuming fewer calories than you are burning. If you are following a diet that does not involve counting calories, then it is hard to know whether you *are* consuming fewer calories than you are burning, and that can make losing weight more difficult.

As an example, we saw a diet where you count 'points' (not calories). That might be a simple way of dieting, and the 'points' might even broadly tally with calories, but things may not work out well. Pasta has no points on that particular diet. So if you really like pasta, you could eat a lot of it, stay within your limit of points, but eat a lot of calories (without even knowing it) and put weight on.

Or you may be following a diet that specifies foods that are forbidden, or foods that can be eaten only at certain times, or foods that can only be eaten in certain combinations, etc. But again, whatever the system is, the success will depend on how many calories you are eating, and if you don't know what calories you are eating, you are at a disadvantage. If the diet stops working for you, it is hard to discover *why* and, more importantly, what you need to do to return to losing weight.

So the problem with diets that are not based on calorie counting is that they will succeed only if their 'system' restricts your calorie intake. And it's pretty obvious that you usually will not be given calorie information on non-calorie-counting diets. The only way you *will* know your calories is if you work them out yourself, and in that case you may as well follow a calorie-counting diet!

What we have both found (and heard from others) is that calorie counting and recording is reliable, flexible, straightforward, and often successful in the long term. However, there will be people who have followed other types of diet, lost a lot of weight, and kept it off – dieting is a personal subject, and almost anything is possible. So if you are strongly attracted to a diet where all you eat before midday is fish fingers and all you eat after midday is pork chops and passion fruit, we suggest that you give it a go. If it doesn't work out, you could always come back and try calorie counting instead – no hard feelings!

To finish off this slice, here is yet another benefit of counting and recording calories. The benefit is related to something we have already mentioned in the book – that to lose a pound of fat, you need a calorie deficit of about 3,500 calories. It is true that the figure of 3,500 calories is a broad approximation and will vary from person to person, but it is good enough to give you an idea of how much weight you might realistically lose by achieving a particular calorie deficit. If you are not counting calories, you won't know what your calorie deficit is and so what is a realistic weight loss for you. And being realistic is important! For example, if your total calorie deficit every week is 500 calories, then you should only expect to lose the occasional pound, and not three pounds every week. It is having unrealistic ideas of what you 'should' lose that can make you fed up and give up.

# Slice 9

# Understand the relationship between calories consumed and burned

As we have already seen, whether you are losing weight or maintaining weight, you need to control two things:
• how many calories you consume (both eating and drinking), and
• how many calories you burn.

If you consume **more** calories than you burn, you will put on weight.
If you consume **fewer** calories than you burn, you will lose weight.
If you consume **the same** calories as you burn, your weight will stay the same.

All of those results are certain to happen – it's just simple biology. However, our bodies are extremely complicated machines, and the results will probably not happen immediately or nice and gradually. They will probably happen in fits and starts, *but they will happen*!

Much of this book is about how to control the calories we consume and the calories we burn, but this particular slice is about why controlling the calories we consume is *much more important* than controlling the calories we burn. That may be surprising to read, because you have probably heard people say something like 'I had a giant meal out with a bottle of wine, then we stopped for a kebab on the way home – whoops! I'll be hitting the gym tomorrow!' You can certainly get the impression that overeating and overdrinking can be fixed by exercising. And some people take it a step further and don't work too hard at controlling what they eat because they know that they spend a lot of time at the gym or swimming or pounding the streets running.

Unfortunately, the bald truth is that nearly everyone who loses weight or maintains a loss does so thanks mainly to controlling what they consume – with just a little help from controlling what they burn by exercising. Why is that? It is simply because it takes a lot of exercise to work off a small amount of food and drink. A lot more than most of us would guess. How much exercise it takes varies with each of us because it depends on our sex, weight, height, age, etc. Let's look at examples in some chat time.

## CHAT TIME

CAROLINE: *It is useful to understand the relative importance of controlling calories consumed and calories burned. Here's one example – lunch today. What did you have?*

STEVE: *I had one cheese sandwich, an apple, and a small glass of orange juice.*

CAROLINE: *That's quite a modest little lunch, not much more than a snack for some people. Do you know how many calories that was?*

STEVE: *Yes, it's about 500 calories.*

CAROLINE: *I know that your exercise is mostly walking, so how much walking do you think it would take to burn off that small meal?*

STEVE: *It's hard to say, but 500 calories is not many, so I think maybe an hour's walk at the most.*

CAROLINE (tapping at the computer): *It's two hours. Even if you ran, you would have to be running for the best part of an hour.*

STEVE: *Oh dear! What about swimming?*

CAROLINE (tappity): *It's still an hour if it's gentle swimming. And it would be gentle, wouldn't it?*

STEVE: *Yes, I'm not much of a swimmer. So how long would it take you to burn off the same lunch?*

CAROLINE (tappity): *Hmmm, I thought so. Because I am smaller, lighter, and a woman, exercise doesn't burn as many calories as it does for you. To work off the same meal, I would have to walk for three hours at your pace, or jog for an hour and a half (or swim for a similar time).*

STEVE: *That is some serious exercise! I suppose we could burn it off more quickly with vigorous exercise.*

CAROLINE: *Yes, I just worked that out. You could burn it off with forty minutes of intensive skipping, or fifty minutes for me. But now we come up against another problem – realistically, what sort of exercise can we do?*

STEVE: *The simple answer is not that sort! We don't have the time, or probably the required fitness, for such vigorous exercise.*

CAROLINE: *And it seems to make sense that people who do undertake intense exercise are generally not struggling to lose or maintain their weight, so they will probably not read our book. Most people who will read it will be in the same boat as we are – they do not (and often cannot) undertake vigorous and prolonged exercise, but they are ordinary women and men who are struggling to control their weight.*

STEVE: *So for many people, exercise comes down mainly to walking. We have been thinking about a 500-calorie lunch, but if we had a big calorific meal with a few drinks, we would be looking at very long walks indeed – at least twenty-five miles. So obviously neither of us can realistically work off a big meal by walking.*

CAROLINE: *True. So although exercise is a help, the most important part of our weight loss is controlling what we consume. As the old saying goes, 'You can't outrun a bad diet.'*

STEVE: *Yes, I like that one! I suppose that both of us already knew that weight loss depends more on diet than exercise. But what I find really interesting is that we are experienced dieters and maintainers, even writing a book on the subject, but we are still surprised to find how much more important diet is than exercise.*

CAROLINE: *True, although we know that we mustn't ignore exercise either. There is more and more evidence that even small amounts of exercise are good for your overall health. And any exercise builds at least some muscle, and muscles burn calories, even when you are asleep.* [We will look at how to increase exercise in slice 23.]

There is another really good reason to focus on learning to control the calories you consume rather than those that you burn. You can do a lot of damage very quickly if you don't control what you consume. Just on the spur of the moment it can seem like a great idea for dieters to eat a big meal (often after having a few drinks), but an hour later the damage is done – they have taken on board 2,000 calories or more. But it is very rare (let's be honest – probably unknown) to go out on Saturday night, have a big meal and a few drinks, and suddenly get an irresistible urge to get your trainers on and walk for eight hours.

So it's calories consumed that should concern us most of all, and that's why much of our book is about calories consumed. But, unfortunately, there is something else you need to understand about calories consumed, and that is that **the more your diet succeeds, the fewer calories you need to consume to keep your weight loss going at the same rate.** Let's look at why that is with some more chat time. Steve talked to Jane, a dieter of fairly average weight and height for a woman.

### CHAT TIME

*STEVE: Thanks for helping me with this, Jane. To begin, can you let me know your weight, age, height, and how active you are?*

*JANE: Not much, then! OK, I weigh 11 st 2 lb, I am forty-one, my height is 5' 3", and I'd say I was moderately active, but not to the point of playing sport.*

*STEVE (tapping at the computer): Thank you ... err ... I make that that you need to consume about 2,000 calories a day to stay at the same weight.*

*JANE: Yes, that seems about right. I certainly need to eat fewer than 2,000 calories a day to have much hope of losing weight. I think you said you were going to tell me how my calorie allowance changes as my weight changes.*

*STEVE: Oh yes, I have my trusty computer. What did you*

*weigh when you started your diet?*

*JANE: I've just celebrated a loss of three stone! So I started at 14 st 2 lb.*

*STEVE: Well done! Let me see (tappity, tappity) ... when you started, you would have stayed at that same weight on 2,250 calories a day, as opposed to your current 2,000.*

*JANE: That's a big difference! And I suppose that when I reach my target weight of 9 st 2 lb, my calorie allowance to stay at that weight will be even smaller than my calorie allowance right now.*

*STEVE: Exactly – as you lose more weight, your daily calorie allowance will continue to fall. But, to look on the bright side, on the day that you hit your 9 st 2 lb goal, you are no longer trying to lose weight, and so your daily calorie allowance will increase a little.*

*JANE: Somehow I think that 'little' increase won't be enough to mean I can go back to eating what I did before – if I did, is it true that I'd put all the weight back on again?*

*STEVE: Yes! And that important understanding is what will help you maintain your weight.*

*JANE: Oh well, it will be worth it to stay at my healthy target weight!*

*STEVE: That's certainly what I've found.*

Although we didn't cover it in the chat time, Jane did ask Steve whether there was any truth in something she had heard – that you need to consume fewer calories as you get older. Caroline and Steve had a brief chat about this.

### CHAT TIME

*CAROLINE: A lot of people do put on weight as they get older, and they often say that it's because their slowing metabolism makes controlling weight more difficult (impossible, even). Can you dig out your computer and figure out how age really affects weight loss?* [Metabolism means the processes in the body that keep us alive and our organs working properly.]

*STEVE: We saw that Jane's calorie allowance fell by 250 a day when she lost three stone. Although metabolism indeed slows with age, her age won't make a difference of 250 calories for years – (tappity, tappity) forty years, in fact!*

*CAROLINE: Wow! So while getting older will mean your calorie allowance is a little lower as time goes on, it's not really a big factor.*

*STEVE: Exactly. What you eat, and even your activity levels, will make much more difference.*

*CAROLINE: And you are an excellent example of this – you lost all of your weight starting at age sixty-one, so it looks as if this 'I can't lose weight because I am older' thing may be a bit of an excuse!*

This has been something of a complicated slice. But where we have arrived at is:
• **It is more important to focus on your calories consumed than on your calories burned.**
• **As your weight falls, the calories you need to consume falls too.**

The result of these two together is that as your dieting success continues, it becomes ever harder to lose more weight. If you want to continue losing weight at the same rate, you will therefore need to (1) consume fewer calories or (2) burn more calories by doing more exercise. Both of these are usually doable, as we will discuss in slices 13 and 23.

But as time goes by, depending on – for example – how much you want to lose, you may find that you do not want to consume fewer and fewer calories. In that case, the option of burning more calories by exercise may become more attractive.

Eventually, if all goes well, you will arrive at your target weight, and you will then be at your lowest daily calorie allowance. But the good news is that the only reason you will manage to arrive at that target weight is that *you will have got used to a new eating regime,* and it should not come as a shock as you move into maintenance. But more about that later!

# Slice 10

## Decide on your approach to social eating events

Many people find that it is easiest to stick to their calorie allowance (or to any other diet system they might be following) when they have a perfectly normal day. The challenges come when their usual routine changes, even if it's in a nice way. Some typical challenges are:

• **When you eat with friends and family, either at somebody's house or at a pub or restaurant.** In these situations, people who are trying to stick to their diets often hear kindly remarks, such as 'It's only for one day' or 'Never mind, what does it matter?' or 'You're doing so well, a day off won't hurt' or 'Calories don't count on your birthday.' Or, unfortunately, they might also hear less kindly remarks, such as 'You're being a spoilsport' or 'You're souring the mood by refusing to eat and drink like the rest of us' or 'Are you trying to make it look as if you've got more self-control than we have?'

• **When your work means you have to spend time away from home or you have to entertain business contacts.** In some ways, both of these situations can be even more difficult challenges than with friends and family. You may have little or no choice of whether you can say 'no' to the challenge, you may have little or no choice of what you can eat or drink, and you may even worry that your job prospects will suffer.

• **When you realise that doing what is expected will not help your diet.** A good example of such a challenge is when people (maybe friends or builders) are coming to visit and you 'have to' provide tea, coffee, biscuits, and cake for them. There seems to be no social pressure to provide apples or celery! Most people greatly dislike the idea that they are acting unsociably, and so they give in to such social expectations and join in eating what they have provided. Or, even if they resist that, they now have those provisions in the house to eat later.

It is tempting to think of these (and other) challenging situations as reasons to ditch the diet for the day, or even for longer. The question, therefore, is whether it is possible to lose weight and keep it off while continuing to have a good social and work life. Obviously, the answer must be yes! Otherwise everyone who was sociable or had a job involving being away from home or ever had builders in would be overweight.

But we believe that it is important, even before your diet starts, to think about what sort of events in your life are going to cause problems with your weight loss or maintenance plans. Then you need to beware of seeing such events as situations beyond your control. If you think that you will 'have to' consume more calories than you want to on your diet, then you are very likely going to struggle a lot to lose weight and to maintain that weight loss.

It is extremely useful if you can work out a way to make sure you get maximum enjoyment from the event, the company, and the food (yes, that too) *and* control calories at the same time. If you can do that, then you will enjoy yourself, feel good afterwards, and find losing weight or maintaining that loss over the long term much easier. And that is what it is all about.

We are all different, and we all have our own social lives, work situations, work colleagues, friends, and families. So you need to work out your own solutions, and slice 22 will help you to do that difficult task. For now, just to illustrate how different people can need different solutions to their social 'problems', let's have a look at some chat time about our own approaches.

### CHAT TIME

*CAROLINE: I think it's been easier for you to handle the difficulties involved in dieting and socialising.*

*STEVE: Maybe it has been in a way. A lot of my life is spent working at home. But then we also go away quite a lot to work as musicians, and that is when we do most of our socialising. Oh, and also I see my family rarely, other than my lovely wife, of course.*

*CAROLINE: That's all quite an unusual situation. How did you decide you were going to handle these periods of being away and socialising?*

*STEVE: I decided, right from the start, that I was going to be completely honest with everyone and tell them that I had a lot of weight to lose and that it had to work. I told everyone I knew that they were going to have to accept a different version of me – a version where I was going to be tough about what I ate and drank, and I was not going to be swayed.*

*CAROLINE: That sounds difficult. Did it work?*

*STEVE: Almost entirely, yes. There were a couple of experiences where I had to be firm, and then people accepted it. And just one person was slightly sulky about it, but my health was more important to me than one person – a person I didn't know very well anyway. How did you manage?*

*CAROLINE: I don't go away for work very much. But I have a family I am regularly in touch with, and I have a busy social life where food and shared meals feature highly.*

*STEVE: Did you also think about how you were going to handle your social eating events?*

*CAROLINE: Yes, but not as much as you did. I don't think I was quite as strong and blunt with people as you were. I suppose I was more worried about offending people. But I did resolve that I would be much more careful in these difficult eating situations.*

*STEVE: And did that more softly-softly approach work?*

*CAROLINE: I would say so, yes. Without my coming out and saying that I was going to be careful and would not be swayed, I think most people got the message. You could say that I was quietly firm!*

So we both thought about how we would plan for social and work eating events and, in our different ways, we felt comfortable with the conclusions we came to, and our experiences were pretty good. Everyone has to look at their own lives and figure out how they are going to address this challenge and make their conclusions work for them. What is key is to see it as a winnable challenge for the canny dieter rather than an excuse to give up the diet!

As we said above, slice 22 contains more detail about the ways in which the challenges can be tackled.

# Slice 11

# Get support from somebody

Dieting is a difficult journey, and it can be a lonely one as well. But our own experiences, and everything we have read on the subject, suggest that getting help in this dieting game increases the chances of success. So we strongly recommend that you line up some suitable support even before your weight-loss journey begins.

Getting 'support' sounds nice, but what do we mean by it? You *can* get help from reading books or watching TV or videos, but most people prefer the help of another human being. Human beings can give advice about what to do (and what not to do), but they can also give encouragement, especially when things are not going well.

You may get support from something like a diet organisation (either at meetings or on an online forum) or – if you can find one – a professional diet helper. But, and often even more useful, there can be more informal sources of support such as (starting with those who may be sitting next to you right now) your partner, another family member, or a friend. For convenience, from now on, we are going to refer to such an informal helper as a 'diet coach'.

Your diet coach does not have to know a lot about dieting and doesn't need to be following a diet, but they do need to be friendly and they do need to be enthusiastic to help you. What they need to do is:
• Be encouraging, especially when things are not going well, for example, when you have been trying hard but your weight is on a plateau.
• Be eager to hear about your dieting plans and how you are sticking to those plans.
• Be able to point out – tactfully – when you are going off the rails for some reason. This can be tricky because it is easy and pleasant to tell someone they are doing really well, but it takes a real friend to tell them they are not!

Finding the right person as a diet coach can be difficult. Your nearest and dearest might be perfect, but they also might *not* be – for example, there are plenty of tales of partners who are not supportive because, for various reasons, they want their other half to stay just the way they are.

But when you do find the right diet coach, it is extremely helpful. Quite apart from having someone to buoy you up when you are down, you will begin to feel accountable to them. This is a fancy term but an important one. If you feel 'accountable' to your diet coach, it means that you are more careful about how you diet, because you do not want to tell your diet coach any bad news. You can see how important it is to find the right person for the job! You need someone who you like and trust, but also someone who you don't want to tell bad news to. Let's look at some chat time where we describe our own experiences of being diet coaches.

### CHAT TIME

STEVE: *We've been one another's diet coaches for nearly three years. But how did it start?*

CAROLINE: *I think it was when we wrote a blog together about some aspect of weight loss, and we shared one another's detailed information about what we had eaten.*

STEVE: *Oh yes, we were only sharing information, but we actually both lost weight in the two weeks of the study.*

CAROLINE: *Because we felt accountable to one another. Remember?*

STEVE: *Ah, yes, I remember. And I also remember that I didn't really believe this 'accountability' stuff at the start. But ...*

CAROLINE: *Yes, go on ...*

STEVE: *... err, in the end, I saw that it was true. And, OK, you were right and I was wrong! After that, we started referring to one another as diet coaches, and we grew into the roles over the weeks and months.*

CAROLINE: *I think we have settled into a fairly robust version of diet coaching, and we are both comfortable with fearlessly pointing out the errors in the ways of the other.*

STEVE: *That's true. I wouldn't say that either of us is thick-skinned, but we have both seen the benefits of hearing the point of view of the other.*

CAROLINE: *And a key point has been that we are completely honest with each other. We've even found that living a long drive from one another is not a problem – it seems to work fine via email. I think it goes to show that getting the right personality combination is all that really matters.*

# The Weight Maintenance Manual
### how to achieve and maintain
### your ideal weight

The four parts of The Weight Maintenance Manual are:

Part 1: What you need to understand
so you can lose weight successfully

Part 2: The actions that you need to take
so you can reach your target weight

Part 3: What you need to understand
so you can maintain your target weight forever

Part 4: The actions that you need to take
so you can maintain your target weight forever

# Welcome to

# Part 2

# The actions that
# you need to take
# so you can lose
# weight successfully

# Slice 12

# Learn to problem-solve

After all the understanding you acquired in part 1 of the book, we are now in part 2, where we get into the serious business of looking at *what you actually need to do* in order to lose weight. In this slice, we are going to look at how you can learn to problem-solve. But before we do that – guess what? We need to explain just a little more, this time about what we mean by problem-solving and why it's so important. We understand that you may be impatient to get on with knowing what to do to lose weight, but please just bear with us for another couple of minutes:

• **There are always problems in trying to lose weight.** You may remember from slice 1 that we spelt out why weight loss is so difficult. We said that weight loss can be difficult because of evolution, the way our brains work, our emotions, time pressures, choosing a diet that is inappropriate for you, and, last but not least, the diet industry. Basically, it's a nasty cocktail of difficulties, and most people are going to experience one or more of those difficulties on their weight-loss journey.

• **It's easy to give up in the face of problems.** People can find that when there are problems in their normal routine, they feel like putting their diets aside – you may have heard (or used yourself) the expression 'life got in the way'. And often 'putting the diet aside' turns into giving up entirely.

• **Dieting problems are personal to you.** Once you come across one of those near-inevitable problems, there's something else that can make it difficult to carry on with a diet – it is hard to get any useful advice from others. That's because every single person on the planet is different; for example, we have different backgrounds, different likes and dislikes, different attitudes, and different body characteristics. Not only that, but everybody finds themselves in a different situation in life; for example, we have different families, different circles of friends, different (or no) jobs, and different places where we live. General advice such as 'eat fewer calories' may help, but you may also receive advice such as 'eat more fibre' when you know you cannot do that because of a medical condition you have.

Putting all this together, we hope you see that (1) trying to lose weight usually involves problems, (2) problems often lead to giving up, and (3) advice you receive may be of little use because we are all different. And we hope you also see that it is no wonder that so many diets fail – but there is a way out of this difficult situation. You can do your own problem-solving to figure out what you need to do. We think that this is probably the most important point in the whole book. It may seem daunting, but don't worry. Keep reading. We can help!

**You can learn to problem-solve, and here's how**
Let's start with some chat time concerning a real example of diet problem-solving.

*CHAT TIME*

*STEVE: When I started my diet, I wanted to cook more meals from scratch.*

*CAROLINE: That is certainly something useful to do, from a nutrition and a weight-loss point of view. Did you do it?*

*STEVE: No, not at first.*

*CAROLINE: Why not?*

*STEVE: Well, I knew it was a good idea, but I didn't have time to do all the preparation of vegetables, salad, and fruit before meals.*

*CAROLINE: A lot of people say that. So what did you do?*

*STEVE: I had a think about whether I could prep ingredients at other times. I thought that maybe I could do it once a week, maybe on Saturday morning, and put everything in the freezer.*

*CAROLINE: And did you?*

*STEVE: Quite often yes, although sometimes I was busy on Saturday morning. But then I realised that it didn't have to be Saturday morning; sometimes I could do it at other times of the week. And then it occurred to me that I was prepping some raw ingredients where I didn't need to put in so much effort.*

*CAROLINE: Don't tell me – you were peeling mushrooms.*

*STEVE: Err ... yes. So I stopped doing that, and then I stopped peeling carrots, potatoes, apples, and cucumber. I just washed and sliced them, so I was saving time as well as getting more fibre and more flavour.*

*CAROLINE: Were you and Ann both happy with this change to unpeeled ingredients?*

*STEVE: Usually, yes. We weren't too keen on unpeeled beetroot at first, but we did want to save the time in peeling it, so we persevered and quickly got used to having unpeeled beetroot. But then I hit another snag.*

*CAROLINE: What was that?*

*STEVE: The freezer was packed with ingredients, but I still had the problem of finding the time to actually cook the meals.*

*CAROLINE: Did you start to change your mind about cooking from scratch at that point?*

*STEVE: No, I didn't. I asked Ann whether we could have our evening meal later, to give me time to cook it from scratch. She didn't want to do that; what do you think she suggested?*

*CAROLINE: A slow cooker?*

*STEVE: Err ... yes (again)! In fact, we had two slow cookers at the back of one of the kitchen cupboards. I did wonder whether you could still get slow cooker recipes, but it took all of five minutes to find lots of useful websites, and then even more websites once I realised that they also go under the name of 'crockpot'.*

*CAROLINE: And then, of course, if you made a slow cookerful one day, you could eat just some of it and freeze the rest. Another time-saver. So what you achieved was eating more nutritiously, eating fewer calories, and saving time.*

*STEVE: Yes, indeed. A win-win-win!*

This all happened soon after the start of Steve's diet, and he quickly got into the habit of prepping and cooking in bulk, and hence eating fewer (sometimes calorific and salty) ready meals. There was a lot of problem-solving going on in that chat time, so let's highlight some of it.

Steve was clear what his problem was – he didn't have time to prepare vegetables, salad, and fruit before each meal. He figured out a solution prepping everything once a week, but when that didn't quite work out for Saturday mornings, he didn't give up, but he kept looking to do things in a different way. He was flexible, so although he didn't know much about slow cookers, he quickly found out all about them. He was open to other opportunities, realising that he could also save time by not peeling some ingredients. Also, and crucially, he never got discouraged – he did not use the setbacks as reasons why he could not solve his problem, but just kept looking for solutions. And finally, he found some good solutions and made them work – he has carried on for years with the same approach to finding the time to cook from scratch.

This all worked well for Steve for several reasons. These reasons include that his job allows him to be flexible about what he does when, that the household is just his wife and himself, and that they are both happy to eat slow-cooked meals, eat vegetable skins, and freeze ingredients and indeed whole meals. **But these may not be true for you** – as we said above, we are all different, and we all need to be able to do our own problem-solving to figure out what we need to do – to figure out our own 'rules'.

But although we are all different, we believe that there are some general problem-solving steps that can be applied to all of us. They are:

1. Be clear about what your problem is.
2. Think about what solution there may be to your problem.
3. If you see a snag with your solution, don't dismiss it too quickly. Be flexible about how you might do things a little differently so your solution still works.
4. If you are sure that your solution can't work, don't let yourself get discouraged.
5. Think about another way of solving your problem. Again, don't be quick to reject your solution! How could you adjust it?
6. Don't give up. Keep repeating steps 3, 4, and 5 until you find a solution that you think will work.
7. Once you have a solution that you think might work, try hard to *make* it work. Be determined. Give it a really good try and, if necessary, adjust your solution as you go along.
8. Despite trying hard to make it work, if your solution clearly *won't* work, repeat steps 3, 4, and 5 yet again.

9. Be determined that you will find a solution that works for you – keep trying; don't get fed up and give up!

If you find that you are not all that determined or that you are getting discouraged, then we suggest that you pause for a time and consider two questions: (1) exactly why do you want to lose weight and (2) what benefits will you have from losing weight?

If you can't answer these questions, then you are going to have a really hard time keeping to your diet – because of a lack of motivation. If you carry on trying to follow a diet, the risk is that you will do it in a half-hearted way, and half-hearted dieting is usually doomed to failure. We therefore strongly suggest that you re-read our slice on motivation (slice 3) before you continue.

We have to re-emphasise that solutions need to be personal to *you*. People will often give you a solution – but that is *their* solution, which works for *them*. If you try their solution and find it doesn't work, then please don't get fed up and give up – it is unlikely that someone's else's solution will work completely (or at all) for you. It will probably need adjustment to fit your own exact circumstance. We all need to make our own solutions by our own problem-solving, and the better we do that, the better our chances of getting to our target weight and keeping at that weight forever.

Let's now have some more chat time, including some examples of tailoring problem-solving. We hope that it will show you what an individual business diet problem-solving can be, and perhaps give you some ideas to start solving your own problems.

### *CHAT TIME*

*CAROLINE: First of all, I have often read how difficult it can be to diet for people who work nights, with the disruption of 'normal' patterns of sleeping and eating.*

*STEVE: Yes. I don't remember ever seeing advice about that, which is quite surprising because there are about three million night-shift workers in the UK.*

*CAROLINE: So that's a first good example – if you work nights, you will have to figure out yourself what works for you in terms of what to eat and when to eat it.*

*STEVE: A second example is the question of whether it is*

*possible to go on holiday and not to gain weight. I know that you are particularly interested in this subject.*

*CAROLINE: Yes, I am. Largely because it is a problem I have often come up against myself over the years! The approach I have settled on is to ask myself which foods and drinks are really essential to make my holiday enjoyable – and happily have those. And reduce (or even cut out entirely) those that are not essential to my holiday enjoyment.*

*STEVE: And, of course, what is essential and not essential is different for everyone.*

*CAROLINE: Exactly. And that's why there is no point in giving people 'rules' about what they 'must' avoid on holiday. Everyone has to figure it out for themselves.*

*STEVE: A third question for people who want to lose weight is how can they lose weight when they have to cook for a family?*

*CAROLINE: Oh yes. This could be a thousand-page book all on its own, simply because every family is different.*

*STEVE: My family, as I've said before, comprises two adults, both of whom are unfussy eaters. Cooking for that family is pretty easy.*

*CAROLINE: While some families comprise a woman who is trying to lose weight, who does the cooking for an ever-hungry man and two children, and they all want to eat at different times and eat something different.*

*STEVE: I always wondered how it was possible to lose weight in that environment.*

*CAROLINE: It's difficult. But if that's the situation you're in and you are highly motivated to lose weight, you can do it. But it is going to be particularly difficult unless you problem-solve how to do it and arrive at your own solutions.*

*STEVE: And now the fourth example. When I started to lose weight, I also started doing some exercise – simple walking. I worked my way up to 10,000 steps a day. But I always envied people who could do 20,000 or more.*

*CAROLINE: Yes, I remember that. What did you do in the end?*

*STEVE: I problem-solved how I could fit 20,000 steps into a day, but I realised that everyone I had heard of who managed it either didn't have a job or they had a job that involved a lot of steps (a postman, for example). So this particular problem-solving finished with my deciding that I could not do 20,000 steps regularly.*

*CAROLINE: So you gave up?*

*STEVE: As if! No – I was flexible. I saw that my problem was not so much trying to do 20,000 steps but, instead, it was trying to do more exercise. So I decided to keep my steps around 10,000 but top it up with some brisk running.*

*CAROLINE: That's a good example. Life is rarely perfect, and sometimes problem-solving leads to something good, but not wonderful. So you ended up with less exercise than you had hoped, but it was better than before, and you could still fit it into your working day.*

Before leaving this slice, we have two final thoughts about problem-solving. The first is that the solution(s) you arrive at should involve food, drink, and exercise, all of which you really enjoy. Or, at the very least, that you can *learn* to enjoy. You are setting out to lose weight and keep it off forever, not to punish yourself for the rest of your life. The day you think it's a life sentence is the day you will give up, and that is one of the reasons that so many people succeed in losing weight for a short time, then give up and regain their lost weight.

The second thought is that when you are looking for things you really like, remember you're not stuck with them for years. If you try eating cauliflower 'rice' rather than the real thing, you might not like it. Or if you have a go at dance classes, that might take up too much time. So just stop them. Have a think and try something else. You need to be flexible and you need to be determined!

We don't usually finish slices with a summary, but this slice is so important that we will do it here, as follows. It's inevitable that, sooner or later, your diet will come up against problems. You can either use every problem as a reason/excuse to give up the diet for a few days (or even a few weeks at Christmas!) or you can learn to problem-solve to find your own solution, and so make it easier for you to lose weight and keep the weight off.

# Slice 13

# Reduce your calories consumed

Many people say that to lose weight, you just have to consume less and move more. We believe that ourselves, except for one slippery little word – 'just'. Yes, the key to losing weight is to consume less and move more, but the word 'just' gives the impression that it is easy to do that. For the vast majority of people it is *not* easy – if it was so easy, why do we have a huge global obesity problem?

We certainly believe that the key to losing weight is to consume less and move more, but we also believe that it's difficult to do those things. In order to make the successful journey from being overweight to being someone who manages to maintain a healthy weight forever, you need to understand an awful lot more than simply the need to consume less and move more. Quite apart from anything else, in this book we have just two slices dealing directly with 'consume less' and two with 'move more' – so what on earth are the other forty-eight about?! We didn't write them for fun, you know! Having got that off our chests, here is the first 'consume less' slice (we'll get to 'move more' a little later).

Let's begin by saying that **in order to consume less, you need to take in fewer calories**. You may well read that and think that it is blindingly obvious, but not everyone is so sure. There are systems of losing weight that do not directly concern themselves with calories. Some systems, for example, are based on consuming foods in certain combinations. Other systems are based on consuming foods that are measured on a points system. And there are many, many others. For some people, these systems may succeed. But, as we said in the preamble, one of our strongest beliefs is that the only way to lose weight is to consume fewer calories than your body burns and that the most effective and reliable way of consuming fewer calories – by far – is to count those calories.

We are not going to tell you that counting 'points', for example, won't work. It might. But our own experience is of losing and maintaining weight by counting calories, and that is what we are writing about in our book. We do know a little about other systems, but if those systems appeal to you, you would be much better off reading something written by experts in those systems.

In fact, our calorie-counting system is easy to describe.

- Set yourself a daily allowance of calories you can consume – an allowance that has been worked out so that you will lose weight.
- Every day, keep a running total of how many calories you have consumed.
- If you consume no more than your daily allowance of calories, you will lose weight.

Simple. Amazingly simple. So let's look now in more detail at both calorie allowances and calories consumed.

## Set yourself a daily allowance of calories

A daily allowance of calories you can consume, so that you will lose weight, is just like a budget of money you can afford to spend. In the same way as you can spend up to your budget, you can 'spend' calories up to your calorie allowance.

The big question is 'What daily calorie allowance do I need to set in order to lose the weight I want to lose?' That allowance depends on many things, such as your gender, your age, your current weight, your height, your level of physical activity, and how quickly you want to lose the weight. Oh yes, and the calculation is often all in metric, and it needs some real mathematics to work it out. But the good news is that there are apps that will work it all out for you. As we have already said, we used *Nutracheck*, which does the calculation, but if you google 'how many calories are needed in order to lose weight?', you'll find the calculation elsewhere on the internet.

## Keep a running total of calories consumed

Using our preferred system, once you have a daily calorie allowance, every day you need to weigh what you eat and drink, so you can keep track of how many calories you have already consumed that day. Once you know that, you will know how many calories you have left, and you can use that information to know what else you can eat and drink that day.

Way back in the last century, we had to look up the calorific value of all of our food and drink, then write the calories down in a (paper) food diary. Fortunately, the calorific value of pretty much everything is now available online, as are systems to keep track of daily calories. We suspect that one of the reasons our own diets have finally succeeded after decades of yo-yoing is the availability of internet assistance. Again, *Nutracheck* has been our assistance of choice, but other internet-based products are available.

In a nutshell, that's it – set a calorie allowance and consume within that allowance, and you will lose weight. But, of course, the devil is in the detail. Caroline's friend Zoe has a keen eye for spotting problems, so let's see some chat time involving the two of them.

## CHAT TIME

*ZOE: I like the idea of calorie allowances and keeping a running total throughout the day. But – how can I put this? – constant calorie counting looks like a big pain. Is it really worth the effort?*

*CAROLINE: Like most things, it gets easier and easier the more you do it. The more you do it, the more you learn how many calories there are in foods you often eat. Steve and I reckon that calorie recording takes us about five minutes every day.*

*ZOE: Couldn't I just estimate?*

*CAROLINE: It seems like a good idea but, for most people, it just doesn't work. There seems to be a powerful human urge to underestimate what we are consuming. And if you underestimate the calories in very high-calorie foods, such as butter or pasta, you will have a big problem. If you think you could be the one in a thousand who can make estimating work, you could always try it. But be prepared to be disappointed!*

*ZOE: OK, I'm convinced; I don't usually think of myself as one in a thousand. On another point, can I eat what I want within my calorie allowance?*

*CAROLINE: Here's some good news – yes! It's like once you have spent money on essentials (on rent or the mortgage, for example), then you can spend whatever is left on anything you like. It's the same with calories, except here you are even freer – there is nothing that is 'essential' to consume, so it is entirely up to you what you spend your calories on. You don't have to deprive yourself. In fact, you mustn't deprive yourself because it increases the risk that you get fed up and give up.*

ZOE: I do like chocolate. Could I include a lot of it in my calories for the day?

CAROLINE: That's funny, we had exactly the same question concerning chocolate from somebody else! [That was Theresa in the slice 8 chat time.] And the answer is yes! You could spend all of your calories for the day on chocolate if you wanted – as long as the calories are within your calorie allowance, you will lose weight. Mind you, there is also the matter of your general health! An all-chocolate diet would be most unhealthy, and before long, you would probably feel ill and hungry. But if your one and only goal was to lose weight, it would work. It would be extremely difficult – you would probably need to be one in a million.

ZOE: Ah. I see the odds are stacked against me again. But you mention healthy eating. Can't I lose weight just by eating healthily?

CAROLINE: In theory you could, but it's risky. You need to be careful not to confuse 'healthy' foods with low-calorie foods. There are lots of foods that are nutritious but calorific – salmon, nuts, quinoa, sweet potato, and avocado as examples. It might be surprising that salmon, gram for gram, is more calorific than a rump steak, nuts are more calorific than cheese, quinoa is more calorific than rice, sweet potato is more calorific than white potato, and be particularly careful of avocado – it looks a bit like a pear, but it is five times more calorific! It's true that some 'healthy' foods contain important nutrients, but it's calories that matter more when losing weight – it's impossible to be healthy if you are fat but well nourished! Unless you were one in a hundred million!

ZOE: OK, well, one last point. You haven't mentioned alcohol yet. I do like a couple of glasses of white wine in the evening. Is that OK as long as they are within my calorie allowance? From what you've said, it sounds like the answer is 'yes'.

CAROLINE: I would say that the answer is 'yes, sort of'. Again, it is fine in theory, but alcoholic drinks are high in calories, and so need to be treated with care. For example, a small (125 ml) glass of white wine is 100 calories, and that can be gone in *a couple of enthusiastic gulps. Not only that, but alcohol has the effect of sapping your willpower, so it can seem like a good idea to have another few glasses and then stop off at the chippy on the way home. And not even chocolate has that effect. But Steve often points out that he lost ten stone having two pints every night – of beer, not white wine! However, Steve is a 6' 1" man, with a much higher calorie allowance than most women. So, as I say, drinking wine is possible but needs care.*

There are two other points we would like to touch on about the daily calorie allowance and counting system.

**It is important not to fool yourself.** Several experiments have shown (as Caroline mentioned in the chat time) that people routinely understate the calories they have consumed. But people also tend to overstate the calories they have burned – a double whammy. If people do that, it is likely that they will not lose weight at the rate they expect or at all. They may even put weight on. So it is important to treat the task seriously – weigh everything you consume, and record everything accurately. The more you do that, the better your weight-loss journey will go.

**Resist the temptation to 'take out an overdraft'.** In other words, don't overeat now, promising yourself that you will consume less tomorrow, next week, or next year. Our experience (of ourselves and of others) is that paying back such an overdraft rarely happens. It is much better to consume less now in order to lose some weight *before* some overeating that you know is coming up.

We are now going to move on to a subject that we think is of great importance to weight loss and weight maintenance. It is closely related to reducing calories consumed, and it is:

**Small permanent changes**
Both of us see small permanent changes (or SPCs for short) as critical to our weight loss and subsequent weight maintenance success.

Many diets and diet books are about a drastic change in your pattern of eating or exercise (or both). Let's say it works – you stick to the drastic action, you lose weight, and you achieve your target weight. Now what? This is often when the trouble starts. Losing weight by taking drastic action and making big changes to your eating and drinking (calories consumed) or increases in your exercise (calories burned) may have worked well for a few weeks or months. But if these drastic changes are not sustainable forever (and maintenance is more or less just that – forever), it is going to be unlikely you will maintain that weight loss. As you will have gathered by now, we think maintenance of weight loss is the really important bit.

So unless there is a particularly good reason to lose weight quickly, it is usually a better idea to use a gentler weight-loss approach than a more brutal fast-as-possible approach. If you do it gently, you will probably acquire good eating and exercise habits – habits you will be happy to follow for years to come. If you can keep going with those habits, you have a good chance of staying around your target weight. Maybe even forever. A good example of this better approach is not to severely restrict or even cut out whole groups of foods, but rather to make a lot of small changes – and these are our small permanent changes. SPCs add up, often surprisingly, and the total can make a big difference to your ease of losing weight, and especially to maintaining that weight loss forever.

### CHAT TIME

*CAROLINE: Just as a bit of background, where did this idea of SPCs come from?*

*STEVE: I'm always reluctant to claim invention of an idea, because people can sometimes pop up to say that they first thought of it thirty years before. But the first I heard of it was when Ann and I talked about it at breakfast in a hotel.*

*CAROLINE: Not such an obvious place to get a good idea about losing weight!*

*STEVE: No, indeed. But it started when I had skimmed milk on my cereal rather than semi-skimmed. It's not a big difference in calories, but we have breakfast at that hotel chain about forty times a year, and the breakfast is always identical. So, even in my head, I could figure out what difference it would make to my weight. The answer was about half a pound in a year.*

*CAROLINE: That's not much! There must be more than that to justify all the time you spend talking about SPCs!*

*STEVE: You're right. I immediately started to think about*

*other small tweaks I could make – tweaks that I wouldn't really notice but would add up. As I remember, the tweaks I came up with were to cut out having dried fruit sprinkled on the cereal, to have a slightly smaller bowl of cereal, and to eat a plain yogurt rather than a vanilla-flavoured one. The total of all of those was nearly five pounds a year.*

*CAROLINE: Five pounds a year is well worth having! And, of course, once those changes become habit and you eat in that slightly different way, then just these tiny changes – at breakfast, and only forty days a year – would make quite a difference. And a permanent difference. Over ten years it would add up to fifty pounds – not far off four stone!*

*STEVE: I am certainly a big fan of the idea of SPCs, and I try to keep thinking of new ones. I even keep a list of SPCs.*

*CAROLINE: Oh yes, I seem to remember your list. I've got a feeling you're going to read it out to me!*

*STEVE: As you mention it, yes. But I've only got the first page with me – it starts with the four hotel breakfast ideas, then there's a further eight:*
- *Skimmed milk on cereal rather than semi-skimmed.*
- *Less dried fruit on cereal.*
- *Smaller bowl of cereal or porridge.*
- *Plain yogurt rather than flavoured.*
- *Soya yoghurt rather than dairy yoghurt.*
- *Fewer nuts or seeds in salad.*
- *Increase in vegetables, salad, and fruit.*
- *Smaller portions of carbohydrates such as rice, pasta, potatoes, and bread.*
- *Even smaller portions of butter, spreads, or cream.*
- *Reduction of size or frequency of snacks.*
- *Less alcohol.*
- *Fewer biscuits, cakes, and chocolate.*

It is worth saying that although Steve's list is entirely one of food and drink, the idea of SPCs can also apply to exercise. In addition, we have both made small permanent changes to *how we think about things*. As examples, (1) we have moved away from using food as a reward, (2) we worry less about what others think of what we eat, and (3) we use smaller plates and bowls. So the idea of SPCs is quite a flexible one.

Remember from slice 12 that we are all different and that we all need to problem-solve to find our own solutions. So although Steve's twelve SPCs in the chat time suit him, those food-and-drink SPCs do not all suit Caroline, who has her own, slightly different list. For example, Caroline's list includes the use of spray oil and (usually) low-calorie dressing rather than the 'full-fat' version. Your SPCs will probably be different again.

Your diet is more likely to succeed if you can think of your own SPCs, so your weight loss is based on choices involving little or no deprivation. And then you may reach the tipping point beyond which weight loss (and, later, weight maintenance) becomes easier – almost inevitable. But to get to that wonderful point, you do need to figure out which SPCs suit *you*.

We have four last thoughts on SPCs:

• If you are not sure whether a change is worth making, have a rough guess at the calories you will save in a year – every 3,500 calories is a pound off. This will make it much more real to you.
• Maybe using SPCs is what (at least some) 'naturally slim' people do, even if they are not aware of it. Perhaps such people make hundreds of small calorie-saving decisions every day of their lives, so it's almost inevitable that they are lean.
• Thinking about SPCs and making them part of your life is the exact opposite of fad dieting. Fad diets are about big attention-grabbing changes, and they almost never work in the long term. SPCs are about small unimportant-looking changes, which all add up to a big effect with every possibility of permanent success.
• We said earlier that as your weight reduces, your body burns fewer calories. So thinking up more and more SPCs helps to counteract that unfortunate tendency of our bodies and is useful in keeping our weight loss going. We will return to this idea later – when we look at managing calories consumed in maintenance (slice 39).

# Slice 14

# Change what you eat
# and change how you cook

We've already said that losing weight is a difficult business and that it is very unlikely that you will succeed if you do more or less what you have always done. An old saying we like a lot is:

**If you do what you always did, you'll get what you always got**

It might be an annoying little sentence, but it's true! And we particularly like it in its dieting form:

**If you eat what you always ate,
you'll weigh what you always weighed**

There are only two tools you have in order to stop eating exactly what you have always eaten:
• Eat the same foods that you have always eaten, but less of them.
• Eat different foods.
Spoiler alert! You will probably want to do some of each, but let's just look at them one at a time:

**Eat the same foods that you have always eaten, but less of them**
A lot of people do this. They like what they eat, and they cannot imagine eating in any other way. For example, they may not like vegetables, and they are not going to start eating vegetables now. Some people are, anyway, limited in what they can eat because they have a food intolerance or other medical condition. If, for whatever reason, you are not going to eat anything different, then you have only one possibility – eating less. This is called 'portion control' and is widely recommended and widely practised. In fact, it is so widely practised that many people are convinced that it is the only possible way to lose weight.

The difficulty we have with portion control is that there is a risk that you will get hungry, and if people are hungry, there is the added risk that they will binge eat to stop the hunger. There are things you can try, to deal with your hunger (see slice 19), and they might work for you, but we feel that portion control is best used alongside the other tool:

## Eat different foods

The idea of this is to make changes to *what* you eat rather than to make changes to *how much* you eat. What you are looking for are foods that are lower in calories than those you have been eating, and the very best result is to find foods that weigh a lot but are low in calories. Foods like that are said to have low calorie density, and they are good news, *because it is more the weight of the food that stops you feeling hungry,* not *the calories in it.*

As an example, if you ate 100 calories of cooked pasta, that would weigh 70 g – a pretty small portion. Instead, if you ate 100 calories of boiled potatoes, that would weigh 130 g – a medium portion. But if you ate 100 calories of steamed red cabbage, that would weigh an enormous 700 g, which would keep you full for hours.

Our message in this is probably clear – if you don't already, start eating a lot of foods that are low calorie-dense. A search of the internet for 'low calorie-dense foods' will give you a huge amount of information about which foods are low calorie-dense and which foods are high calorie-dense. But even before looking at the information, you may have guessed that the answer is:

• There are good guys – the ones that fill you up and are fairly low in calories, such as salad, vegetables, and fruit.
• There are bad guys – the ones that don't fill you up much but are high in calories, such as chocolate, nuts, crisps, butter, and oil.
• There are in-between guys, including potatoes, pasta, rice, beans, lentils, meat, fish, bread, and cereal.

In a perfect world, your problems are now over. You just need to stock up on all the good guys, you won't be eating many calories, and you'll feel full. But it's not a perfect world because, even as you are reading this, you may be thinking that you don't like salad, vegetables, and fruit. What do you do about that? This much is for sure: whatever you eat, you have to enjoy it. You will never get to your ideal weight and then maintain that weight forever (and, remember, that's the whole idea) if you have to eat foods you don't like. Food is one of the great pleasures of life for most of us – it has to be a pleasure, and it has to stay a pleasure!

The answer that both of us found to this was to deliberately set out to *learn to like* low calorie-dense foods where we didn't like them already. This is a personal thing, and we can't give you any rules to follow – some people are interested in trying new foods, but others call themselves 'fussy' or 'picky' eaters and absolutely cannot or will not touch anything new. The problem for people who are reluctant to try new foods is that if a lot of what they eat is high in calories (typically high in sugar or fat or both), then they are going to find it difficult to lose weight. Their main tool is going to be portion control, which, as we said before, can easily lead to hunger.

So we can't give you any rules, but we can give you some thoughts (followed up with some chat time):

• If you are keen to lose weight, it is a good idea to explore other foods.
• If you do not like a food, you may come to enjoy it if you keep trying it again and again. Remember what we said about habits in slice 2?
• You might not like a food presented in one way, but try it another way. For example, a lot of people dislike celery, but what some really dislike is raw celery. If they tried it made into a soup or cooked at the same time as onions in a curry, they might come to like it. It's easy to play this game, given the number of recipes available on the internet!
• Foods can be totally different when combined with others in different ways – in other words, how you cook foods may make them more palatable to you, even if you are a picky eater.

If you manage to find and enjoy a big range of low calorie-dense foods, you are well on the way to successful weight loss and successful maintenance. We think that our own successes are largely down to our choice of food and how we cook it, and so we are going to spend some time now looking at a chat where we talked about what we had done and continued to do.

### CHAT TIME

*CAROLINE: Let's begin by talking about the ingredients we use in our cooking. After you.*

*STEVE: I suppose that the ingredients I use were originally driven by my decision to continue eating big meals – all of my previous diets failed because they made me hungry, and I dislike feeling hungry.*

*CAROLINE: Oh yes, I've seen your meals – big portions of low-calorie foods.*

*STEVE: That's right. I eat large portions of foods such as lettuce, celery, and green beans, but small portions of foods such as cheese, garlic bread, and chips. In fact, this is good fun – I really like cooking, and it's a daily challenge to cook big and interesting meals containing few calories. That's not your approach, is it?*

*CAROLINE: No, not really. I am happier with a more traditional diet, where I still have some calorific foods, such as bread, pasta, rice, couscous, and potatoes. I just keep my portions small.*

*STEVE: That's interesting because that sort of portion control doesn't work well for me, and I have several decades of failed diets behind me to prove the point.*

*CAROLINE: And once more, we see that we are all different! It's another example of how we all have to problem-solve to find our own solutions – in this case, how much we are going to use portion control and how much we are going to eat different foods. In my case I've used both, because I also added in foods that I had rarely, if ever, eaten before.*

*STEVE: Which foods were they? I thought you already had wide tastes in food.*

*CAROLINE: That's true, but they were fairly unusual things, such as persimmon, kidney, and red quinoa.*

*STEVE: Fascinating! But why did you do that if you were good at portion control?*

*CAROLINE: It was to make my meals more interesting. I think that's an important part of a weight-reduction diet – to maintain the pleasure of eating.*

*STEVE: It's the same for me – I certainly wanted some different foods to give me more variety. Because I actually stopped eating quite a lot of high-calorie foods (pasta, for example) for the whole time I was losing weight.*

*CAROLINE: You do have quite an all-or-nothing approach. You know that it's not usually recommended to eliminate foods from your diet altogether, don't you?*

*STEVE: Yes, I do know, but I can be a bit of a rebel! In any case, the addition of (for me) many new and interesting salad, fruit, and vegetable items more than compensated for giving up some foods entirely. And I have found that one of the pleasures of looking for lower-calorie foods when shopping is that some of them are delicious, and I enjoy them for their taste alone – it's just a bonus that they are low in calories.*

*CAROLINE: It's certainly important to keep an open mind. We have both discovered what we thought would be impossible – enjoyable non-alcoholic beer, which is a health win-win (no alcohol and few calories)!*

*STEVE: And I have grown to love some of the non-dairy milks, yoghurts, and puddings – lower in calories and fat than their dairy equivalents and delicious.*

*CAROLINE: It is well worth everyone trying new foods from time to time to see what substitutions work for them. We have touched on what we eat, but what about how we cook it?*

*STEVE: I keep it simple and cook without any oil or fat at all, making liberal use of lemon and lime juice. I tried that as an experiment at first and found that some things were slightly odd, but I persevered until I found dishes Ann and I liked that did not involve oil or fat. That meant that we saved many thousands of calories a year.*

*CAROLINE: Just as I remembered – your approach was rather more extreme than mine! I am certainly careful with oils and fats in my cooking – I never splosh them on, and I am a big fan of spray oil! I also use low-fat substitutes, such as low-calorie sauces where available, and measure those carefully as well. And I use small amounts of low-calorie dressing on my salads.*

*STEVE: An interesting chat – we are both successful dieters, even though there are significant differences in what we eat and how we cook.*

We hope that chat illustrated how we both stuck to the principle of using more and more low calorie-dense foods and cooking them in interesting ways. But we also hope that we got across that we did it differently – there is no right or wrong here. Everyone enjoys eating differently, and we all have to find our own way of enjoying our food.

Also, we don't want you to lose sight of what we said earlier in the slice – changing foods is a great tool, but portion control still has its part to play. To really enjoy eating, most people want a balanced diet, and, while you may have come to love eating lots of low-calorie vegetables, you may still want lasagne with garlic bread from time to time. And it's *then* that we all need to be good at portion control. We may not even bother weighing our pile of low-calorie vegetables, but it is a good idea to use some careful portion control on that lasagne and garlic bread – because we know that we can eat a thousand calories of that pretty quickly!

# Slice 15

# Change the way you shop

There is a close connection between shopping and eating. If you eat meals at home, you will need to shop for the ingredients, except for unusual circumstances such as if all your meals are prepared by someone else or if you live off the land. And if you haven't shopped in the right way, you may not be able to cook well or eat well – and losing weight will be harder. Shopping is therefore at the heart of dieting, and this slice is all about how dieters can shop better in order to diet better.

Our advice, in a nutshell, is don't go shopping without a plan, be sure to make a shopping list, buy only what is on your shopping list, and buy only the *amounts* that are on your shopping list. Let's look at each of these.

**Don't go shopping without having a plan of what you are going to be eating**
Clever shopping begins even before the shopping starts. Thinking ahead about your eating over the next few days is an important part of shopping well. Planning in this way may be a change for you, but it is the modest changes you make (as in so many other aspects of dieting) that will pave the way for losing weight and maintaining your weight loss.

If you are following the system that we suggested in slice 13 – counting calories and eating within your daily calorie allowance – then the basis of your shopping plan is probably clear already. That basis is that you need to be thinking of what meals you will be having over the next few days. How many meals will you be at home for? How many people are you feeding at each meal? Do you need packed lunches? Then you need to figure out how you will stay within your calorie allowance for those meals, which will probably involve lots of low-calorie foods.

This figuring-out is especially useful if you sometimes undermine your weight loss by grazing (or bingeing) on problem foods outside mealtimes. You won't be surprised to hear that by 'problem foods' we mean high-calorie snack items, typically high in fat and sugar. So we mean foods like chocolate rather than foods like celery, though we're sure that you already knew that! The cheapest and simplest solution is not to buy the problem foods in the first place. That way, if you have the urge to eat (say) chocolate, you can't just go to the cupboard for it – you will have to go out and buy it. That whole delay process allows time for the chocolate urge to subside.

So far, we have talked about planning your eating to include lots of low-calorie ingredients. But you may be thinking that you will have to buy some high-calorie foods for the others in the family. There may be something in that, but it's important to avoid thinking that buying some high-calorie foods means that *all* of your dieting ambitions go out of the window. Avoid thinking that you may as well just stock up on everything that's high-calorie and ignore the foods that are going to help you to achieve your target weight.

If the others in your family are old enough to buy the high-calorie food for themselves, let them do it. But if they are younger children, then think about the message you send if you buy healthy food for yourself but *continue* to buy unhealthy food for the rest of your family. It looks as if you are saying that you are concerned about your own health, but you are OK with letting your children eat unhealthily and probably gain weight. We're sorry to put this so bluntly, but we think that you would be setting a better example by limiting your children's eating of unhealthy food.

You may be thinking at this point that being firm about serving healthy food to the other people in your household is a nice idea but would simply be impossible. Perhaps, for example, you are the only one in your family who wants to lose weight, and maybe you are outnumbered by assertive, always-hungry but always-lean people who demand large high-calorie meals. There are unlimited family situations in which you might find yourself, so, as much as we'd love to give you the solution, only you have the answers to your own specific problems. What we *can* do, however, is suggest that you look back to slice 12, where we talked about how to problem-solve to find solutions that work for you. It may give you some ideas.

**Make a shopping list**
Once you have a clear idea of your eating plans for the week, now is the time to make a shopping list. We think it is important to make a written list, whether it's on a scrap of paper or on your phone. Carrying the list in your head carries the risk of forgetting something, and it is easy to forget that what you needed was a large swede but quite easy to 'remember' that you had a need for chocolate cake.

Also important is to have the amounts on the list. It's easy to buy too much 'to be on the safe side', but that can easily lead to eating too much (as we will see shortly).

The ideas we are trying to get across here apply equally to online shopping. In fact, it can be better for the dieter to shop online because the online shopping list that you post on the shop's website has to be exact – you can't put 'something for dinner on Tuesday', which you *can* do on a paper shopping list. You are also obliged to put down the number of each item you need, although it still doesn't stop you from erring 'on the safe side'. For simplicity here, however, we are going to assume that you are making your own list and going out shopping.

Having made the shopping list, the next important step is to remember to take it with you! Pieces of paper and even phones can be forgotten, and you will have to try to remember what you were supposed to buy. Then you will have the swede/chocolate cake issue, but many times over.

**Buy only what is on your shopping list**
You planned your meals and made a shopping list. Now you're in the shop. It may already be too late to take our first piece of advice (so remember it for next time!), but don't be hungry when you go shopping. Being hungry is likely to make you buy foods that are not on your list and more likely to buy what *is* on your list, but in larger quantities. And we have never met anyone who reacts to shopping while being hungry by buying too many Brussels sprouts. More likely, for some strange reason, people buy too many doughnuts or four-cheese pizzas.

In fact, whether it is caused by being hungry or not, it isn't a good idea to depart from your shopping list except for obvious mistakes (such as forgetting the bleach). You might prefer to shop spontaneously, but please bear in mind that sticking to a list is another useful change to make in order to help your diet objectives. If you don't buy it, you won't eat it!

People often depart from their shopping list because they see foods in the shop that they did not have on their shopping list. We are thinking here of foods that will tempt you, which once again are unlikely to be Brussels sprouts. The trick is simply not to go into the areas of the shop where the tempting foods live – it's so much easier to resist temptation if it is not staring you in the face!

If you have remarkably strong willpower, you may wonder why our advice here is necessary. But if (1) you are someone who has ever eaten something 'that you didn't really mean to eat', or (2) you have ever eaten something from the fridge 'just because you opened the door', or (3) you have ever eaten a second chocolate bar 'because it called out to you', then this is good evidence that your willpower may not be all it might be! And it would probably be useful to your diet to take this section seriously.

**Buy only the *amounts* that are on your shopping list**
Even if you have mastered the skill of buying only what is on your shopping list (and well done if you have), you still need to master the skill of buying only the *number* of each item that your list said to buy. It probably goes without saying that this second skill is more important for more calorific items – but we will drive the point home, just in case! No harm is likely to come to your diet if your list said to buy one head of celery but you bought three. It's a different story if your list said to buy a 2,000-calorie chocolate cake for a special celebration but you bought three of *them*.

This subject of buying the right amount is important, and we are now going to introduce an idea that we, and many others, have found helpful.

*CHAT TIME*

*STEVE: There are literally hundreds of millions of words that have been spoken (and written) about dieting, so it's rare to find an idea that has not been talked about already. But I am pleased to say that we are now going to talk about your brand new idea – the idea of Sprogonomics!*

*CAROLINE: Quite an introduction! But credit where credit is due – it was you who dreamed up the term 'Sprogonomics', based on 'Sprog' – my username on the Nutracheck site that we have already mentioned.*

*STEVE: I think a good way into Sprogonomics is to give an example. I particularly like the example you often use – if your daily calorie allowance means you can eat just a single bar of chocolate but you see that you can buy two bars in a two-for-the-price-of-one (BOGOF) offer, Sprogonomics tells you not to buy the two bars.*

*CAROLINE: Spot on! In theory you might eat just one bar and keep the other one for another day, but here in the real world, this is unlikely to happen. More likely is that you will eat both bars. In money terms it's a good deal, because each bar is half price. But in dieting terms it is bad, because you will be eating more calories than you wanted to, and so you will be harming your weight-loss plans.*

*STEVE: And that's it in a nutshell – Sprogonomics is a principle where decisions about food are made much more because of the benefit to your weight than because of the benefit to your bank balance. So the chocolate bar example goes against Sprogonomics because it only makes sense in money terms, not in dieting terms. And the more we thought about your idea, the more we saw shops and restaurants everywhere going against Sprogonomics.*

*CAROLINE: Yes, there is a good example in many restaurants. If two people are in a restaurant and each wants a single 250 ml glass of wine costing £5 (so a total of £10), then it is common to be offered a whole 750 ml bottle for (say) £12. That is clearly going against Sprogonomics – in money terms it makes some sort of sense, but you are going to drink more than you intended to drink, which means that you are going to consume more calories than you intended to consume.*

After that Sprogonomics interlude, perhaps it is now clear why we recommend having a shopping list that includes the amounts to be bought and buying just those amounts – without 'taking advantage of' special offers such as BOGOFs. Generally, we steer clear of special offers because we think of them as traps, which are trying to trick us into buying more of something that will hamper our weight-loss ambitions.

Essentially you need to be cautious! Remember that supermarkets are not our friends – they are big businesses working in a cutthroat market, and they want us to take a lot of things off the shelves and pay at the till. They do not care about our health and wellbeing. And they do not care whether we can afford it or not – the only reason they run (for example) BOGOF promotions is to get us to spend more. We often remind ourselves of four little sayings we have come up with to help us remember that shops do not want us to be canny, calorie-conscious shoppers:

- They know that something that looks like a 'bargain' encourages people to buy things they wouldn't otherwise buy (and eat).
- They try to fool you with clever marketing.
- Don't line supermarket coffers and get fat at the same time.
- BOGOF really stands for 'Buying Objectionable Gains Of Fat'!

# Slice 16

# Enjoy your food and eat without guilt

Neither of us made a deliberate decision to become overweight, and you probably didn't either. Nonetheless, we did gain weight, and so (presumably) have you. Nobody is pleased about weighing more than they want to weigh, and sometimes people become cross with themselves about it. This kind of thinking can lead to weight-loss plans that are harsh and hard to keep to. In this slice, we think about a different approach: this is a diet, not a punishment! Ideally, you will never feel guilty again about what you are eating.

By now you will have gathered that our aim for ourselves was not just to lose weight but was (and still is) to lose weight and keep it off for the rest of our lives. The obvious difficulty was that both of us enjoy our food. We like cooking and eating, especially with family and friends, we like eating out, we appreciate a wide variety of foods, we like trying new foods, and we enjoy a glass or two of wine with a good meal in good company.

Neither of us has a special secret supply of willpower, so moving to a lifetime of limited food options without these pleasures was never going to work in the long term (and the long term is what we are interested in). It was important to find a way of eating that we could maintain for life, and, generally, we have succeeded. We have made big changes in what we eat while still regularly enjoying food that is not considered 'diet food'. Zoe wanted to know the secret of our success.

*CHAT TIME*

*ZOE: You seem to keep to a good weight but also to eat some nice food. I have always tried to make my diets quite strict, so that I lose the weight faster.*

*CAROLINE: That's a common approach to dieting. What happens when you try a particularly strict diet? Can you keep to it?*

*ZOE: Yes.*

*CAROLINE: Good. What's the problem, then?*

ZOE: *Well, I can keep to it for a time, but not for long enough. Perhaps I just don't have enough willpower.*

CAROLINE: *What happens after you stop keeping to it?*

ZOE: *I go back on it but try to be a bit stricter to make up for it.*

CAROLINE: *Does that work?*

ZOE: *Not really; the same thing happens again.*

CAROLINE: *It sounds as if a different, not so strict way of dieting might work better for you?*

ZOE: *A diet where I can eat what I like? Bring it on!*

CAROLINE: *We-e-e-ll, it's not quite like that, but a diet where you can eat some of what you like, some of the time! Which also happens to be a diet where you can eat some food that is off-limits on most diets – but where you don't feel guilty or punish yourself. Will that do?*

ZOE: *Yes!*

CAROLINE: *You may have to swap the idea of losing weight fast (but failing) for actually getting to your final weight-loss goal and maintaining that weight for the rest of your life.*

ZOE: *OK, I'm in! Tell me more!*

We'll now have a look at the diet Caroline promised to Zoe. Our two big messages are (1) there are snags in completely cutting out enjoyable high-calorie foods and (2) it's possible to eat anything you like and still stay on your diet.

## Snags in completely cutting out enjoyable high-calorie foods

**Cutting out foods makes them more desirable.** It is a peculiar part of human nature that as soon as something is forbidden, it becomes even more desirable! So making a particular food a rare and special treat makes you yearn for it. That means that trying to eliminate foods you enjoy from your diet is really tricky because as soon as you cut them out, you start to want them even more. And on top of that, the more you try *not* to think about something (such as cream cakes or beer), the more likely it is to come into your mind.

Even if you manage to cut out all these foods in the short term, there is a big danger that you are doing this because you believe that when you have lost the weight, you can bring them all back into your diet. As past experience will probably tell you, that is no way to maintain your hard-earned weight loss. And remember what we said in slice 14 – if you eat what you always ate, you'll weigh what you always weighed!

**Restrictive diets can get boring.** If you are eating only a small range of foods – foods that people tend to think of as 'diet foods' (such as celery) – then it's easy to get bored with them. That's especially true if these are not foods you enjoy. And if you get bored, then is it more likely you will get fed up and give up the diet altogether.

**Restrictive diets can become a vicious circle.** If your diet is full of foods you don't enjoy much and you don't have any foods that you really like, it will be much harder to keep to the diet. When you 'give in' and eat something that is 'off-limits', you will feel cross with yourself. As we saw with Zoe, this can become a vicious circle of trying to be even more strict in your dieting next time with the same results.

**Cutting out all the foods you enjoy can make your diet feel like 'the enemy'.** As thoughtful human beings, we instinctively fight against feeling controlled by anything. If you try and cut out of your diet all the pleasurable foods you enjoy eating, it leads to a feeling of deprivation and of being controlled by your diet. You can even come to see your diet as 'the enemy'. On the other hand, if you make wise choices about what you are eating, you will feel in control of your diet, more 'at peace' with your diet, and you will find it easier to keep on track.

**Feeling guilty about eating something takes the pleasure out of it.** When people eat something that is being 'forbidden' by their diet, they often feel guilty. And when they feel guilty, the pleasure is not as it should be – they tend not to enjoy that 'forbidden' food properly or feel satisfied after eating it. So you get the worst of both worlds; you get all of the calories but not much pleasure. As Steve said in one of his more poetic moments: 'The pleasure has been washed away by the bitter taste of guilt.'

#### It's possible to eat anything you like and still stay on your diet

We have just looked at several snags involved in cutting out enjoyable high-calorie foods. So the obvious question now is how can you eat such things without ruining your diet?

There are three ideas below about how to eat foods that are traditionally off-limits for dieters:

- Choose what matters most to you.
- Plan your meals (and other eating).
- Enjoy eating those foods you like – without guilt.

If you follow these ideas, you can eat without guilt and still lose weight. It is possible to put these ideas into practice in various types of diet but, for us, the inclusion of 'non-diet foods' is one of the areas where calorie counting works particularly well. It makes our three ideas clearer and simpler, and you will lose weight – as long as everything you eat is accounted for in your calories and you are eating fewer calories than your body needs to maintain weight.

**Choose what matters most to you**
We hope that you will not be surprised when we say that you cannot have all of the high-calorie foods you enjoy *and* every time you think you would like them *and* in the quantities you used to have *and* still lose weight! That's the bad news. The *good* news is you can swap around these pleasures and enjoy some of them at any time without feeling guilty and still lose weight – and you might be a little surprised by that! You will still need to make choices about what you eat, how much of it you eat, and how often you eat it, *but you don't have to exclude anything.*

How much leeway you have for these foods depends on both the rest of your diet and your daily calorie allowance. If you are a six-foot man looking to lose ten stone, you will probably have a daily calorie allowance of around 3,000 at the start of your weight loss journey. You can spare a few hundred for (as an example) beer and still eat well.

If, on the other hand, you are a five-foot sedentary woman hoping to lose that last half a stone, to be genuinely slim, you may have a daily calorie allowance of more like 1,400 at the start of your weight loss. If you choose to spend a couple of hundred calories a day on wine and crisps, you may have not much more than 1,000 calories left for the rest of the day. It is possible to do that, be well balanced nutritionally, and also lose weight, but it will be tricky. If you also wanted 400 calories for a nice cheese sandwich at lunchtime and 200 calories for a chocolate snack every day, it would be very difficult to do.

All this means that we need to make choices about what matters most to us in food and drink. A choice we often need to make is about portion size – for example, whether to have a fun-size chocolate bar, not a standard one. Another choice we are often faced with is about frequency – for example, how often can we have alcohol, crisps, or chocolate, where the answer may be not all three on the same day, or all three on Saturday, or any one of many other possibilities. This is highly personal – each one of us has a different list of what food and drink matters most to us, so each one of us has to decide what choices to make. There is a phrase that we both use a lot and has helped us to make these personal choices about what we would like to eat or drink: is it worth the calories?

A final thought here: if you are trying to lose weight fast, especially if you have not got much to lose, you are likely to be following a rather severe and low-calorie plan that is quite restrictive. In that case, you won't have much leeway for making choices. This is one of the many reasons we favour a steady and modest weight loss of a maximum of two pounds a week.

## Plan your meals (and other eating)
If you want to have a glass or two of wine with your evening meal, then record the calories for that wine at the start of the day, so you know what you have left for food. If having something sweet in the evening is important to you, then make sure you have a couple of hundred calories left for it. If lunch isn't lunch without a packet of crisps, then have one, even every day – just make sure you put the relevant calories into your calculations or your diary and work around it.

If you decide that it isn't a good idea to have something that day, then it can be helpful to think that you are delaying having it, rather than depriving yourself. It is useful to say to yourself, 'I'm not having that cake today because I want to keep within calories. I'll plan it in for tomorrow.' Then it feels less of a deprivation. Suddenly you are feeling in control because you are looking forward to something nice rather than being controlled – and deprived of it.

## Enjoy eating those foods you like – without guilt
Finally, we think that deliberately planning to have those higher-calorie foods you want can be a pleasant part of dieting! It can be fun to choose which foods you are going to have and at what times. When you know these foods are a part of your diet and not sinful or a reason to be punished, you can sit down to eat them with pleasure, not guilt.

You can make eating these foods even more enjoyable by using the idea of 'mindfulness' (see slice 19). In the context here, mindfulness means paying close attention to those higher-calorie foods, including noticing their taste and texture. That makes eating them more satisfying and, as a bonus, it means you are less likely to want some more of them immediately afterwards. You have arrived at the point where you are enjoying what you eat without the aftertaste of guilt – delicious!

Just before leaving this slice, you may remember Zoe was enthusiastic to try our idea of a guilt-free diet, eating some of what you like, some of the time. There was a happy ending – we gave her a draft of this book, she followed our thinking pretty closely, including our advice in slice 6 about losing weight steadily, and, at the time of writing, she is maintaining a weight loss of about four stone. Pleasing for Zoe and pleasing for us!

# Slice 17

# Don't use food as a reward

Losing weight is not easy, and dieters are quite rightly pleased when they have had some success. Maybe they lost weight or maybe they stayed the same when they had expected they were going to put weight on. After such an achievement, it is common to want a reward, and there is nothing wrong with that. And the most natural way to reward yourself is with what you may have been missing so much – food! At first sight this seems to be a clever idea – it's a sort of edible and motivational wall chart. Lose weight – reward yourself. What could go wrong?

Let's explore this with some chat time. We know many people who reward themselves with food in this way, so it wasn't difficult to find somebody to talk it through with Caroline.

*CHAT TIME*

*CAROLINE: Hi, Sue!*

*SUE: Hi, Caroline. I'm so pleased! I weighed myself this morning, and I've lost two pounds. Calorie counting works! I'm going to have a couple of chocolate-covered ginger biscuits with my cup of tea this evening to reward myself. I've missed them, because I used to have three every single evening with my cuppa. But I have cut them out since I started calorie counting.*

*CAROLINE: Well done! And if you can afford the calories for this biscuit reward, it sounds like a nice plan.*

*SUE: Yes, I've counted it all up, and the biscuits fit in with my calorie plan. I can't wait!*

*CAROLINE: The only problem I see with this, and I'm so sorry if I seem like a spoilsport, is that to lose weight and keep it off, things have got to change. And one thing that all we dieters need to change is thinking of food as a 'reward' or as a 'treat'.*

*SUE: But what's wrong with that? I've always enjoyed having nice food as a treat.*

CAROLINE: *Having always done it is the trouble – if you always make something into a reward or a treat, it makes it even more desirable to you. So you end up with a really strong link between being pleased about something and eating something sweet, fatty, and calorific. It might not matter much for a quick diet, but that's not what Steve and I are about. We're aiming to help you keep your weight off forever, and in order to achieve that, it's best not to return to previous habits.*

SUE: *Oh. But does that mean I can never have those biscuits again? I really like them.*

CAROLINE: *Certainly you can have them again – you may have heard us say before that this is a diet, not a punishment! But the way to do it is to plan the biscuits into your diet as part of your normal eating rather than as some special reward. And, of course, do plan them into your diet – don't end up eating the whole packet!*

SUE: *OK, that's fair enough. I was beginning to dislike you for a moment there!*

Sue is just one example among many. We see an awful lot of people talking about having a 'treat day' or a 'cheat day' or 'a day off' after – for example – a successful weigh-in. And maybe the above chat makes it clear why it is not a good idea. If it *isn't* clear, allow us to hammer it home! It's because it is all too easy to strengthen the idea that food is extra-special and extra-desirable. That is particularly damaging because the kind of food people have in those situations is nearly always calorific, sweet, and fatty – we have *never* seen anybody rewarding themselves with Brussels sprouts!

Remember, from right back in slice 2, that the more often you do something, the easier it is to do it next time – which is why habits are so difficult to break, especially if there is immediate pleasure in doing it. If Sue rewards her weight loss with a biscuit, she is also making it more likely that she is going to want to have a biscuit next time she feels pleased with herself about something. This is just snatching defeat from the jaws of victory – you've had a big success; now turn it into failure by doing what you had managed to stop yourself from doing. It undermines maintaining in the long term, which cuts right across what we are trying to encourage in this book.

People often argue that they *do* have the willpower to have (say) one nice chocolate-covered ginger biscuit just this once, as a special treat. That might be true, but we think it is unlikely. We have seen so many people whose diets are failing while they are frequently treating themselves to some food as a reward – we think the number of people who can control it is small, and we strongly recommend you not to attempt this feat. Anyone who does have such amazing willpower would probably not have put on weight in the first place!

**So what *can* I use to reward myself?**
We need to make it crystal clear that we are all for rewarding ourselves after achieving something good. Especially if we have achieved something good in our dieting, which, as we never stop saying, is a most difficult task to pull off. Reward yourself – *but just not with food*!

If not food, then what is a good reward? Obviously what is a good reward is a personal choice, but here are some things (in no particular order) that one or both of us use as non-food rewards. We hope they give you some ideas.
• Being pleased with ourselves or 'patting ourselves on the back'. Noting (even writing down) how pleased we are can help us remember the feeling and work towards it another time.
• Perhaps surprisingly, a reward we are not expecting – a surprise reward – is usually even better than one we have planned for ourselves. Good examples of these surprise rewards are when someone comments on our weight loss or a stranger says something about us looking thin. These make us feel really good! It is worth noting them, and both of us write them down so that they are not forgotten.
• Think about things that are easier and more pleasant because we have lost weight. The fit of clothes, for example.
• Small gifts.
• Or maybe bigger gifts. Caroline did think about putting aside a pound coin every time she achieved one of her dieting targets and then using that for some really nice clothes. She hasn't done this one yet because she is not sure that new clothes are a big enough incentive for her. So she has also wondered about building up a holiday fund instead. As we said, it's a personal choice.
• Finally, one from Steve. Neither of us totally approves of this one, because it does involve food. But Steve finds it motivating, and he doesn't always toe the party line in every detail, so let's include it. Steve does not use sweet, fatty, and calorific foods as rewards (good so far!), but he does occasionally reward himself with foods that are expensive,

difficult to prepare or difficult to get hold of where he lives. As examples, dragon fruit and duck.

We will leave this slice with one last thought for you: our experience is that people who automatically think of food when they feel pleased (or disappointed) with themselves are often overweight. And those who *don't* automatically think of food when they feel pleased are often *not* overweight. We know which side of the fence we want to be on!

# Slice 18

# Change the way you deal with surplus food

You shopped according to your plan. You've been eating carefully. How is it possible to end up with surplus food? Here are some possibilities.

• Your shopping plan was good, but you didn't eat everything you bought, and food is left over. There was simply more food than you needed.

• Your shopping plan was maybe not all that good. It included buying some foods that you possibly shouldn't have planned for, and they are left over. What we mean here is buying such things as cake, biscuits, or wine because people are coming round – people such as family, friends, neighbours, or builders.

• Your shopping plan was good, but somebody later gave you something like cake, biscuits, or wine. We use the same examples as above – after all, it's not often that guests arrive armed with a big bag of celery for the host(ess)!

What these have in common is that you are left with food or drink that is surplus to your immediate needs. We'll look at what you might do about your surplus in a minute, but first, let's have a look at what you might do to minimise any surplus next time. There are indeed situations where it's usual to provide refreshments, such as tea, coffee, biscuits, cake, etc. But even if you think that applies to your own situation, it's a good idea to try to reduce any surplus there might be. For example, it could be perfectly OK to offer tea without biscuits. Or not to offer cake *and* biscuits. Or two kinds of cake.

Also, although it's not really relevant to this slice, we can't resist pointing out that just because everyone else is having those calorie-rich refreshments you have provided, that does *not* mean that you have to have them as well!

OK, you did your best to stop a surplus arising, but it has still arisen. **How do you get rid of it?** Many people have a horror of throwing food away, and so they eat the surplus pretty much as quickly as they can. That just damages your diet, so we suggest another approach to your surplus: DO NOT EAT IT. Instead, consider the following possibilities:

• If possible, freeze it for another meal or occasion.
• Take it to a food bank, if you have one nearby.

• Put it out for the birds. It's better for the local wildlife to get overweight than you!

• Throw it in the bin or pour it down the sink.

• Give it to family, friends, neighbours, or builders. Possibly the ones you bought the stuff for or possibly the ones who gave it to you to begin with. If the surplus follows a visit to your house, you could always do what Caroline is particularly good at – tell everyone at the start that you are carefully watching what you eat, and that at the end of the visit, would they please take any surplus home or you will throw it away. As we said, people tend to have a horror of throwing away food and drink, so that threat usually does the trick.

It takes a little courage to learn to dispose of a surplus by giving it away or throwing it away. But just do it, and the habit gets established, and it soon becomes second nature. Your family, friends, and acquaintances will quickly accept it and see it as nothing worse than a mild eccentricity.

But if you can't get rid of the surplus, whatever you do, *don't* eat it just because it cost you money to buy it and you don't want it to go to waste! That is wrong for a good reason: because your decision whether to bin it or eat it *has nothing to do with money*! Don't believe us? Put it this way:

**What if you bin it?** You've spent the money and you are not going to eat it.

**What if you eat it?** You've spent the money and you have eaten calories you know you didn't need to consume.

Whichever you choose to do, you've spent the money, and you will never get it back. So the only difference between binning it or eating it is whether you stick to your diet or damage your diet. So bin it!

Even if you can't get your head around that argument, remember that worrying about money in this situation cuts right across the principle invented by Caroline – Sprogonomics, which we explained in slice 15. As a reminder, Sprogonomics is a weight-control principle where decisions about food are made much more because of the benefit to your weight than because of the benefit to your bank balance. So Sprogonomics also tells you what to do. Altogether now: 'Bin it!'

# Slice 19

# Learn how to manage your hunger

We said earlier in the book that when we lose weight, what we are doing is consuming less fuel than our body needs. The problem is, as all dieters know, that when we eat less than our body needs, we are likely to get hungry! That happens because our bodies are highly sophisticated machines and when we eat less, mechanisms swing into action to prevent us from starving to death.

Evolution is not on the dieter's side: being overweight kills slowly, starving to death kills fast, and the body doesn't want that! The mechanisms do not know or care if we want to lose two stone to be a healthy weight. They simply tell our brains that we are hungry. This is really inconvenient – we want to lose some weight, and our bodies are going to do their best to stop us from losing it by making us feel hungry.

We believe that success in finding some way to manage this hunger is fundamental to success in dieting. If you don't find a way of managing hunger, you will be forced to be hungry a lot of the time. It is possible to live that way, but it is difficult and unpleasant – because satisfying hunger is a strong urge in most forms of life.

In this slice, we are therefore going to look at various aspects of managing your hunger, as follows:
• How to think about hunger
• How to reduce hunger by changing *what* you eat
• How to reduce hunger by changing *how* you eat

**How to think about hunger**
We are going to look at some ideas for managing hunger. But first, we need to recognise that however clever we become at doing that, we will never get rid of hunger pangs entirely. The fundamental urge to eat, especially when dieting (in other words, when undereating), will always be there.

Feeling hungry is unpleasant – even being a bit peckish is not nice – and for most of us, it is a feeling that is easily changed by eating. Food, particularly high-calorie, sweet, fatty food, is readily available in the shops and in workplaces. And it is also available in your home (unless, of course, you have already taken our advice in slice 15!).

If you have always eaten a substantial snack to deal with your hunger and you have felt less hungry afterwards, then you have laid down a strong habit of managing hunger by eating. It is easy to believe that it is the only way to manage hunger – because we rarely try anything else. But now is the time to *try* some other approach! We said, right back at the start of slice 1, that 'Human beings are complicated creatures and those massive brains of ours mean that the way we think about and understand things makes a big difference to what we do.' One element of that is that how we think about hunger has a big impact on achieving our target weight and then maintaining that weight. So let's look at some ways of thinking about hunger that have helped us and may help you.

**Think of hunger as an early warning signal.** Hunger is not a danger sign or an emergency. Think of it more as an early warning signal, in the same way as feeling sleepy is an early warning signal.

Most people will have felt a little sleepy at some time during the day. But few of us drop what we are doing and go to bed at that point (which is, anyway, tricky if you are at work or shopping or driving!). What do you do if you feel sleepy in the day? Usually you notice you feel sleepy, but you get on with what you are doing, and the feeling passes. Sometimes you may do something to help you feel more alert, such as have a cup of coffee or wash your face with cold water. And you might make a mental note that you need an early night or two. But you would be highly unlikely to stop what you are doing and go to bed!

Hunger works in a similar way. You are not going to come to any harm from not doing anything about feeling hungry. Feeling hungry is not dangerous, any more than feeling sleepy is. Next time you feel hungry between meals, ask yourself, 'If this hunger was tiredness, would I go to bed right now? If I wouldn't, why do I need to respond to hunger any differently?' Being hungry is not some crisis that needs to be fixed immediately – you can put up with it until your next meal.

**Think of hunger as a feeling that is not of great importance.** This uses the sleepiness example again. Imagine a day when you've been woken by the alarm but would like to go back to sleep. Rather than doing that, you will often have to drag yourself out of bed and get on with your day. Quite quickly, you'll probably start to feel more awake. The whole experience is not particularly important – it's no big deal.

Think of hunger in the same way. If, say, you have eaten a reasonable meal, but you are not fully satisfied and you still feel hungry – it's no big deal. Just get on with doing something else, and you often stop feeling hungry. And remember: hunger is not dangerous, and it will not do you any harm!

**Think of hunger as burning away your fat.** Imagine that those hunger pangs are simply caused by your diet working. They are nothing more than your excess weight being burned off. Steve liked this one a lot – he enjoyed turning his uncomfortable feeling of hunger into a good feeling of weight being lost.

**Think of hunger as really being thirst.** It is easy to think of hunger pangs being thirst, especially because there is plenty of evidence that it is actually true! If you drink a big glass of something (water is good, as it is also low-calorie!), those 'hunger pangs' often just go away.

### How to reduce hunger by changing *what* you eat
Thinking about hunger in a certain way can work well, but it is also helpful to reduce your feelings of hunger through changes in what you consume. There are ways of eating that make your body feel hungry again soon afterwards and other ways that mean you are likely to feel full for longer – even though you have had the same number of calories.

This may seem strange, but it happens because different foods have different effects on the way your body knows it is full. The canny dieter learns to take advantage of this and eats foods that make them feel less hungry. For most of us it takes a bit of trial and error to find what those foods are for us, but it's worth persevering. Once you know which foods make you less hungry, it will make your weight-loss journey so much easier, and therefore more likely to be successful.

Perhaps a less obvious hunger-reducing idea, but an extremely effective one, is to simply consume more! We need to see some chat time on that.

### CHAT TIME

*STEVE: I am pretty sure that one reason my previous diets have all failed is that I was hungry all the time.*

*CAROLINE: How did you diet before?*

*STEVE: Over the years, I have tried all sorts, but I always had to fight hunger – and when I lost the fight, my weight loss stalled, and I got fed up and gave up.*

*CAROLINE: What has been so different this time?*

*STEVE: I knew from the start, I must find a way of eating that didn't leave me hungry but was also low enough in calories for me to lose weight. I realised I wanted to eat a large quantity of food, but that it needed to be low-calorie food. That led me to eating a lot of vegetables and salad in my lunch and dinner.*

*CAROLINE: It obviously worked well – and that's not surprising, as you were eating in a way that meant your stomach had a lot in it, which sent the 'I'm full' signals to your brain. And all the fibre meant it would have been bulky in your intestines too, so the 'full signals' would have kept going for some time. Great plan!*

*STEVE: How did your eating change on this diet?*

*CAROLINE: I also increased the vegetables and salad – though I worked up to it more slowly. I'd always been pretty good on my five portions a day, but now I generally eat more like ten. But the other big change has been eating much less sweet stuff.*

*STEVE: And that means your blood sugar levels stay much more stable and your hunger isn't triggered by sudden drops in blood sugar levels.*

*CAROLINE: And, like you, I generally find my true hunger is minimal and manageable.*

*STEVE: Another useful tactic, then.*

There are some other points to consider, concerning reducing hunger by changing what you eat. Again, perhaps surprisingly, the points are about eating more, not less.

The first is that if you regularly find you are hungry before the next time to eat, it might be worth considering whether you are eating *enough of the right foods* at your meals. Caroline finds that she benefits from what we might call a 'proper meal' at lunchtime, by which she means some fish and vegetables. That can contain no more calories than a sandwich, but she finds that it's more satisfying and keeps hunger at bay for longer in the afternoons. Steve finds that an enormous bowl of salad for lunch serves the same purpose.

The second is that if you are hungry and pretty sure you are going to have a snack, make it something nutritious and filling, not something sweet. This is helpful because (1) it will keep you full for longer and (2) it is not so immediately rewarding that you will want another one! And if you find yourself thinking 'I don't want soup – I want a biscuit,' then you are probably not hungry at all. In that case, you are either craving something or your hunger is triggered emotionally. We will cover these in slice 20.

And finally, there is a belief (not yet fully substantiated) that not being well-nourished can lead to hunger because your body is trying to get the nourishment it needs. If that is correct, making sure that your diet is well-balanced and nutritious may help to prevent hunger. To be honest, even if this belief turns out to be wrong, it's always good for you to maintain a well-balanced and nutritious diet – even if it doesn't help prevent hunger!

**How to reduce hunger by changing *how* you eat**
Apart from reducing hunger because of what we eat, we can also tackle it by eating in a different way. You might find that frequent small snacks enable you to keep hunger at bay and your meals do not need to be as big. Or you might find that snacks do not affect your hunger at mealtimes at all, but merely add to your daily calorie intake. Something of a theme to this book is that there is an amazing variety in the way our bodies behave, and we have to experiment to find what works for us. So you might like to experiment with the frequency of between-meal snacks and what you eat for those snacks.

Eating in a different way also covers *where* you eat. For example, if you eat in the kitchen, it is not a good idea to continue sitting there after you have finished eating, because there will be other things to eat in the kitchen and you might be tempted to have a little something else. But if you think you might eat something else, even if you don't eat in the kitchen, just do something else – go and have a bath, or maybe go for a walk.

A little more chat time might illustrate some of these points.

*CHAT TIME*

*CAROLINE: I'm always surprised that you never snack at all. Why do you think that is?*

*STEVE: To some extent, I think it's the environment in which I spend most of my time. I usually work in a small office at home, nowhere near the kitchen and with no stocks of food of any kind (biscuits, for example). On rare occasions I wander into the kitchen to make a drink, and then I sometimes pick up an apple. So I do snack a little.*

*CAROLINE: That's interesting because Ann and myself spend much more of our time around our kitchens, and it's easier to just graze, almost without thinking about it. And I work in an office a lot, where there are all the usual 'team biscuits' and 'cakes on birthdays' rituals. There are many more opportunities for Ann and myself to eat things that we didn't intend to. We have no ready answers to this, but you do need to be aware that if you live and work in an environment where snacking is easier to do, you need to be especially careful.*

## Mindfulness

Our final idea concerning how to manage your hunger applies to whatever you consume and in whatever situation you find yourself. That idea is that, whatever you eat, eat it 'mindfully'. Originally part of Buddhist traditions, mindfulness has been practised in the Western world only since about 1970, and its popularity has fluctuated. This is a pity, because it can be a useful skill. Many thick books have been written about mindfulness, and it is a skill that takes many years to learn. We are not able to teach all the subtleties of mindfulness here, but there are two key ways in which mindfulness can help weight loss, and we will briefly look at those. If that whets your appetite, the internet is your friend – in fact, we have just googled 'mindfulness' and had 141,000,000 search results!

One aspect of mindfulness is being aware of what you are feeling and recognising that it is simply a feeling and nothing else. The discussion above about the meaning of feeling hungry and the fact that it is not a danger sign or a crisis is an aspect of mindfulness: you notice what you are feeling and don't need to react to it by eating something.

Another aspect of mindfulness, which is more often mentioned in dieting circles, is 'eating mindfully'. That means to eat, paying close attention to what you are eating. Maybe that seems obvious to you, but if you have ever munched your way through a big bag of crisps in front of the TV, or had a chocolate biscuit, then realised you have eaten the whole packet, or drunk some wine or beer quickly because you were thirsty or simply because it 'evaporated', then you have consumed something 'unmindfully'. You may have been satisfying your hunger or thirst when you started, but, sure as anything, your hunger or thirst was fully satisfied well before you had finished the last crumb or drop. To put it simply, you were consuming calories that you didn't need to consume, and you didn't even notice you were consuming them.

All you need to do is the opposite of consuming 'unmindfully'. In other words, do things like enjoy the aroma, consider how it looks on the plate, notice the sensation of the food in your mouth (temperature, texture, dryness, moistness, creaminess, chewiness), be aware of the sound as you eat it (does it crunch?), and pay close attention to the flavours. You will get more enjoyment out of eating, and you will not be eating without even noticing that's what you are doing.

Eating 'mindfully' is a skill. It's not all that easy to acquire the skill, but it's well worth persevering because eating mindfully is another useful tool on your weight-loss journey and on your maintenance journey.

# Slice 20

# Handle emotional eating

We discussed emotional eating in slice 4, and that included looking at how your body can't tell if there is a *reason* for overeating – it simply stores the surplus calories as fat, whether you've got a good reason or not! So we've got some understanding of emotional eating, but if you are affected by it, we now need to look at the tricky subject of what to do about it – how to handle emotional eating so it doesn't get in the way of your weight-loss plans.

But first, **congratulations**! You have recognised that you sometimes eat emotionally *and* you have made the brave decision that you want to do something about this in order to meet your important goal of becoming (and staying) a healthy weight. You are on your way!

The first and most obvious way to deal with eating too much of the wrong foods because of your emotions is to deal with those emotions in a different way. And again, this is not easy. You may not even be aware of your emotions, or you may be perfectly well aware of them but feel powerless to change them. We are now going to return to the separate categories of spur-of-the-moment emotional eaters and longstanding emotional eaters, which we introduced in slice 4.

**Spur-of-the-moment emotional eaters**
We have already described spur-of-the-moment emotional eaters – as people who eat in quick response to emotions, situations, or other people. If this is you, and if the source of such emotion is unclear to you, the first step is to pay attention to the point at which you experience the emotion. Is there a situation or person or mood that seems to trigger the emotion? And there may be more than one trigger, because if you have learned that this behaviour works for you, you will most likely use it for more than one thing. The more you can recognise the pattern of your behaviour, the easier it is to deal with.

Over time, you may recognise that you respond to a particular emotion by overeating. The most effective solution (whether when losing weight or in the longer term – when you are maintaining) is to find some way to make these emotions trouble you less. Here are two examples:

• Do you always overeat when you have a row with your partner (and this happens often enough for you to put on weight)? Then it might make sense to look at your relationship as well as your eating.

• Do you often dig into the big stock of biscuits you keep in your desk drawer when working late at the office, all on your own? Then it might make sense to try to rearrange your working life so that you can go home earlier – even if you have to carry on working once you get home.

You may be able to work out some of these on your own. Sometimes you may need the involvement of other people – friends, relatives, or perhaps health professionals or counsellors.

Everybody's emotional eating is different, but we are going to look at five techniques that can be helpful in combating the urge to eat in response to an emotion.

## Describe the emotion

It can be enormously helpful to teach yourself to identify and describe (or put a name to) the emotions you feel when you overeat. This helps you notice that what you are feeling is *not* hunger but something else entirely.

As soon as you notice that, you are opening the door to responding to the desire to eat in a different way. Why would you eat chocolate in response to your boss being unfair to you? How will that help? Will she be kinder to you if you weigh more? Will being fatter mean you no longer expect people to treat you properly? As soon as you look at it this way, it becomes a little easier to resist eating as a solution, but the first step of describing the emotion is key.

There is another benefit of describing your emotions – in doing it, you are *respecting* what you are feeling, not *avoiding* what you are feeling. You might deserve sympathy and support for whatever you are feeling, and there is no harm in giving that sympathy to yourself. Furthermore, the acknowledgement of an emotion can sometimes make it less powerful, less strong, and less painful. It is also a good way of helping you stop and think about what you are feeling rather than moving immediately to use food in an attempt to take away the feeling.

Like so much that is worthwhile in life, describing what you are feeling takes a little practice! And you probably won't get it right first time. If, however, the next time you find yourself overeating because of an emotion, you think, 'Oh no, I didn't remember to describe what I was feeling,' then this is a step in the right direction – although it might not seem like it at the time. Go back in your mind and ask yourself, 'When could I have described or named it?' If you practise doing this in your head (even after the event), it makes it more likely you'll notice it next time!

## Delay eating

There are two major benefits of simply delaying eating as a way of solving emotional eating. The **first** is that it gives you time to manage the emotion differently, so you may not feel the need to eat as strongly. The **second** is to do with the food itself. If what you are most aware of is a desire to eat ice cream, and nothing else will do, then it will be easier to resist at the moment of crisis. If you say to yourself, 'In an hour, when I am calmer, if I really want some ice cream, I can have a measured bowlful.' It's well worth trying this out for yourself – notice what happens to the urge to eat when you don't immediately give in to it.

## Distract yourself

Imagine that something has happened that has perhaps upset or angered you, and you are heading for the fridge. Then you remember: 'I'm not hungry; I'm furious' (helpfully describing the emotion as well). You tell yourself, 'I'm not going to eat just because I am angry – if I want something to eat in an hour, I'll have something.' And now you have an hour to fill; how are you going to fill it?

Again, planning helps! It is well worth thinking in advance what might help in this way. Contacting other people can be helpful. Or possibly going for a walk or a run or taking some other kind of exercise. Taking yourself away from the food helps, maybe to have a bath or shower or to clean your teeth. Doing something incompatible with eating helps, such as painting your toenails, playing a musical instrument, or doing some kind of craft or hobby. Be aware that watching TV or reading is rarely a strong enough distraction, but they might work, especially if you do them in a different room from the food.

Make your own list of distractions for emergencies. When you get an emergency, work down your list. If it's long enough, working down your list will probably take you an hour – a perfect distraction!

## Eat something else instead

If you feel that you are not going to be able to manage any delay, and you *must* eat something, an extraordinarily helpful tactic is to eat something that is much lower in calories than whatever you had in mind. Not many people seem to try this trick, but we both do it often and heartily recommend it!

If Caroline is angry, she likes something with a good crunch. Usually, what she really wants is a biscuit, but in an emergency, eating celery with a smear of marmite often works well. If, on the other hand, Caroline is sad or anxious, she likes something warm and sweet. What she probably wants is treacle pudding and custard, but, in this case, she finds that drinking a cup of low-calorie hot chocolate can take the edge off things. These reasonably good alternatives do far less harm to her weight.

Of course, celery and low-calorie hot chocolate are not as satisfying as biscuits and pudding – but that is a bonus. If the habit of eating when emotional is too hard to break in one step, changing what you eat can be an excellent intermediate step. Earlier in the book we explained that eating sweet and fatty stuff fires off the 'this is nice' parts of your brain; well, the celery and low-calorie drink are far less likely to fire off those parts of your brain. That begins to break the connection between the emotion and the eating.

### Notice how you feel when you eat something in response to an emotion

Finally, if you eat something in response to an emotion, do you enjoy the (probably calorific) food and feel good after it? If not, and as we discussed in slice 16, do you guiltily swallow it down without much pleasure and then feel rotten afterwards? It is worth thinking about how you do feel because if it is the second, you could ask yourself whether such emotional eating has *ever* been a solution to a problem.

### Longstanding emotional eaters

If you think that your overeating and weight gain is, at least in part, due to events in your past, you may be able to work through those events on your own. Although these are not easy issues to deal with, here are some examples of questions you could ask yourself.

• 'Do I want those events in my past to control me and my health while I am trying to diet (and, for that matter, for the rest of my life)?' (Probably not.)

• 'If the events that happened to me had happened to another person, would I think that person deserved their diet to fail, deserved to be overweight, and deserved to be unhealthy for the rest of their life?' (Very unlikely.)

• 'If the events in my past were of an intimate nature and I now want to avoid unwanted attention, is becoming overweight by overeating really the best way to avoid attention?' (Probably not. There will be better ways to achieve that.)

If you are trying to lose weight but you are a long-term yo-yo dieter, it is especially worth asking yourself how you can deal with *other* matters in your life. Because, oddly, however important losing weight is, it does only two things: it improves your health prospects and it means you get to wear smaller clothes. So if your weight gain is a response to other difficulties in your life, unfortunately, losing weight isn't going to solve them. If those other difficulties are still there, you remain at risk of beginning the cycle all over again.

As we said above, these are not easy issues. It is certainly possible to just 'power ahead' with losing weight without dealing with these longstanding issues at all, and you may have done so before. But it will be even harder work for you to lose weight and keep it off than it is for people without such longstanding issues. Steve is a good example of someone who powered ahead, albeit with a less traumatic issue. He was brought up to finish everything on his plate, has never addressed that issue, and still finishes everything now. This can't help his dieting, but he successfully compensates for that by his other dieting techniques. So powering ahead can work, but it needs extra effort.

You may have some success with addressing longstanding issues that cause you to overeat. You may find that the five techniques we discussed when looking at spur-of-the-moment emotional eating are useful. And you may have friends and relatives who are ready, willing, and able to help you. In this difficult area, you may also want the involvement of health professionals or counsellors.

Ideally, of course, you will find the right support *and* you will keep heading towards your goal of losing weight. But even if it takes quite some time to get the support you need, don't give up on losing weight while waiting! The simple fact that you are more aware of the complex issues that we have talked about will help you to separate the emotion from the eating.

# Slice 21

# Learn how to manage cravings

Craving a specific food **right now** is an experience many dieters have. Most dictionaries define cravings as a strong urge or desire for something. The effect of cravings on the dieting ambitions of many people means that they cannot easily be dismissed – even though they are often seen as an 'excuse' by people who do not experience them. Characteristics of a craving include:

• The person with the craving is well aware that they have it.

• Resisting a craving, rather than giving in to it, is particularly difficult.

• Not being able to satisfy a craving leads to feeling anxious, upset, and tense.

• Continually giving in to a craving is usually unhelpful to a diet.

• People with a craving often make a firm resolution to resist in future, only to give in sooner or later.

Whatever the difficulties, however, people who have cravings can and do overcome them. After all, if you go out without any money and a craving for chocolate overcomes you, you are unlikely just to steal a bar of it.

Probably most people would agree that a craving for chocolate, while a powerful urge, is not as powerful as a confirmed smoker's urge to have a cigarette. Also, even the most hardened sixty-a-day smoker has periods when they want a cigarette but don't have one – on public transport, for example. And, what's more, many smokers give up entirely and have to resist powerful urges all day for weeks, months, years, or even forever. Our message is probably clear: if millions of people can stop smoking, then you can manage your consumption of chocolate or whatever your favourite craving is!

**What is the difference between hunger and cravings?**
A craving is sometimes looked at as simple hunger. But, in fact, cravings have almost nothing in common with hunger. Some of the many differences are:

• When **hungry**, if your favourite sandwich isn't available, you'll happily eat an alternative. A **craving** is almost always specific – a packet of crisps will not usually satisfy a chocolate craving.

- **Hunger** tends to build up gradually. A **craving** often arises quite suddenly and is triggered by seeing or thinking about the food that is craved.
- **Hunger** is satisfied with a reasonable amount of food. A **craving** is hard to satisfy and can easily lead to overeating.
- If you are eating to satisfy **hunger**, you will usually eat in much the same way, whether you are alone or in company. Eating to satisfy a **craving** is often done while you are alone.
- Perhaps most importantly, when you are **hungry** and eat a meal, you do not usually feel bad about having eaten it. After eating to satisfy a **craving**, you often feel guilty and unhappy.

So hunger and cravings are significantly different, and it is important to treat them differently. If it *is* a craving you have, what is important is how to manage it so it doesn't hinder your weight-loss progress. Zoe wanted some advice from Caroline on this one!

### CHAT TIME

CAROLINE: *How's the diet going?*

ZOE: *Some days it's fine, but yesterday I was doing well and then in the evening I had such an overwhelming craving for chocolate ... I ended up eating a whole big 100 g bar.*

CAROLINE: *Ouch! What happened?*

ZOE: *I don't really know. I was watching TV, and there was an advert for chocolate and I suddenly really wanted some.*

CAROLINE: *Did you think about resisting the urge or craving?*

ZOE: *For about half a second, then I remembered that I never can resist – it's like an addiction. So into the kitchen I went.*

CAROLINE: *What did you think would happen if you did resist a craving like that?*

ZOE: *But I never do!*

CAROLINE: *So let's think about that. What is the worst thing that could happen if you didn't have chocolate when you craved it?*

ZOE: I'm not sure ...

CAROLINE: Worst case scenario – would it kill you?

ZOE: No! That's just silly! In fact, there have been times in the evening when I haven't had any chocolate in the house, and I certainly wasn't about to get dressed and go to the shop to get some.

CAROLINE: So what are you afraid will happen if you don't satisfy a craving?

ZOE: I'll want it more and more. I might end up eating something else, which will take me over my daily calorie allowance anyway – so I might as well have the chocolate. Perhaps I won't be able to get to sleep for thinking about it, and then tomorrow will be harder at work. I'll be uncomfortable and restless and not enjoy the rest of the evening.

CAROLINE: And what do you think will happen if you do satisfy the craving?

ZOE: I'll feel better.

CAROLINE: And did you feel better after 100 g of chocolate last night?

ZOE: Well, no. I thought I'd have just one square, but that wasn't enough and then, before I knew it, I was on the last square.

CAROLINE: Did you enjoy it?

ZOE: Yes.

CAROLINE: And what happened next?

ZOE: I went back and watched some more TV.

CAROLINE: And what were you thinking about, having eaten a

*big bar of chocolate?*

*ZOE: To be honest, I was feeling really rotten – a bit sick and also cross and fed up with myself. It must have taken me way over calories, and I had been doing so well this week. It's really stupid the way I keep doing this.*

*CAROLINE: Did you enjoy the rest of the evening and sleep well?*

*ZOE: No to both.*

*CAROLINE: OK. So when the craving strikes, you believe that resisting it will feel bad, give you a bad evening, and spoil your sleep. But in fact what you discovered is that not resisting the craving made you feel bad, gave you a bad evening, and spoiled your sleep.*

*ZOE: How strange! I thought that not giving into the craving would be a problem, but what really happened was that giving into it was the problem!*

By the end of that chat time, Zoe realised that the real problem was giving in to her cravings. So now we need to look what to *do* about cravings.

**How to avoid giving in to your cravings**
We have some suggestions:
• **Suggestion 1** is simply to try to avoid getting hungry. It is important to manage your eating through the day so you are not perpetually hungry. It is much easier to manage a craving if you are not also hungry! You may remember from earlier (slice 14) how Steve is good at avoiding hunger because he tends to eat foods that are low in calories; he can eat a lot of them within his calorie allowance, and that full stomach stops him feeling hungry.
• **Suggestion 2** is to create the right environment – one that makes it difficult to satisfy your cravings. The more difficult it is to get to the food you crave, the less likely you are to eat it. You can make it particularly difficult to get to the food you crave by not having it in the house! *And you can achieve that by not buying the food you crave.* If, for some reason, it is essential to have a food that you crave in the house, then make sure it is out of sight. Cravings can be triggered by something you see – the

trigger for Zoe was an advert, but seeing chocolate on the kitchen worktop would probably have the same effect.

• **Suggestion 3** is to notice what is happening and describe it to yourself. Recognise that you are not actually hungry. Some people offer themselves something healthy, which they are *not* craving, to prove to themselves they are not hungry – 'Do I want a hard-boiled egg? No! Then I don't need chocolate!'

• **Suggestion 4** is to ask yourself the same sort of questions that Zoe was asked:

'What do I think will happen if I don't satisfy this craving?'

'What am I worried about?'

'What is the worst that can happen?'

And then remind yourself of what you feel like a few minutes *after* you eat a food you crave. Is this what you want to feel like?

• **Suggestion 5** is that, once you are firm and clear that you don't intend to give in to this craving, you use three of the strategies that we described in slice 20 for avoiding emotional eating. As a quick reminder, those three were (1) to **delay** by telling yourself you are not having it now but can have (some) in a planned way tomorrow when you can work it into your calorie allowance, (2) to **distract** by taking yourself away from the temptation and doing something that occupies your mind (best of all is to choose something you can't do while eating!), and (3) to **eat something else instead** – something that is lower in calories.

• **Suggestion 6** is to think to yourself, 'This is not an irresistible craving; this is a whim, a wish, a want, but not a need.' That may be particularly difficult for you if, like many other people, you tend to describe your cravings as something even stronger than a craving – an addiction. So let's have a look at the difference between the two.

### Do you have an addiction – not 'just' a craving?

An 'addiction' is an inability to stop doing something or using something. Sometimes people desire a specific food so much that they feel that the word 'craving' is not strong enough to describe their desire. Instead they often say that they are 'addicted' to the food. In the case of chocolate, the word 'chocoholic' is used so much that it even appears in reputable dictionaries and has done since the 1960s. But at the time of writing, there is no scientific evidence that it is possible to be addicted to types of food in the way that it is possible to be addicted to (for example) nicotine.

It is important to know that you do not have a true addiction to something like chocolate. You might like chocolate, you might love it, you might crave it, but you are not addicted to it. This really matters because if you believe you have an addiction, you may convince yourself that you have a medical condition over which you have no control. You may then (like Zoe in the chat time) believe that resistance is futile, that you may as well stop fighting it and just eat it!

To use having an 'addiction' as a free pass to eat the subject of your 'addiction' is a real problem. Even if food 'addictions' did exist, you would still need – somehow – to restrict your calorie intake in order to lose weight so that you arrive at your target weight. And not controlling your 'addiction' would harm your plans unless you had a celery 'addiction' (extraordinarily rare in our experience!). Anyway, how could controlling a food 'addiction' be harder than – as we saw earlier – giving up nicotine, which is a certain and medically recognised addiction?

Our advice, therefore, is not to describe any urge to eat something that you like as an 'addiction' (or even as a 'craving'), but merely to say how much you like it. It brings everything into one big category – the category of foods we need to control eating, where nothing has a special status that justifies eating a lot of it.

# Slice 22

# Handle social eating events

People who are trying to lose weight don't usually consume or burn the same number of calories every day. Life for most of us is more varied than that – we go out at weekends, have holidays, and enjoy celebrations with family and friends. In this slice, we are going to call things like that simply 'events'. People often mark these events with increased eating and drinking, and that usually involves increased calories, and that tends to lead to increased body weight.

At the beginning of our own weight-loss journeys we both realised the same – that eating and drinking were woven through our social lives in many ways. Eating with friends and family, whether cooking at home or going out, was one of the great pleasures of our lives. So how on earth was it going to be possible to make being on a diet fit in with a social life? In this slice we are going to share with you seven key 'rules' we made for ourselves, for working through the pleasurable but challenging territory of eating with friends and families. We recommend you give the following 'rules' a try.

- Be wary of forgetting your calories entirely
- Use calorie counting
- Plan for a single event
- Plan for a series of events
- Choose carefully what you eat at social events
- Enjoy what you eat
- Manage social pressures

**Be wary of forgetting your calories entirely**
Whatever the social situation, we always keep calories in mind (although sometimes they are quite far back in our minds!). We often hear people say that they do not want to control their social eating because they feel that 'life is for living' or because they are sure that they will lose any weight gain afterwards. While we happily agree that life is for living, we think that our own social lives are so busy that uncontrolled social eating would be enough to badly affect the progress of our diets. So we do live our lives, always with at least half an eye on what we are eating.

## Use calorie counting

Calorie counting makes many aspects of dieting easier, and navigating your social eating is one of those aspects. As we have said before, calorie counting puts you in charge of what you 'spend' your allowance of calories on, so you can have what you like as long as you count it as part of your total. That means that if you count calories, you know what you are consuming and whether your social eating is getting out of control.

We are not suggesting that it is essential to count the calories of everything that passes your lips on Christmas day – we certainly don't. But if you are a regular calorie counter, you will have learned (roughly) how many calories are in the foods you usually eat. You will therefore know, as you eat a portion of Christmas pudding and brandy butter, that you are spending many hundreds of pleasant calories. And that will give you at least some idea of what weight gain to expect. But that's good! It's much better to know that you will probably see a gain of four pounds and step on the scales and find you were right than it is to have no idea at all, step on the scales, and get a nasty surprise of a gain of four pounds. Why is it better? Because getting a nasty surprise can mean (and you have already heard this often) that you might get fed up and give up.

## Plan for a single event

We love a good plan! This is about planning for a single instance of eating or drinking that you know will not be good for your diet – for example, a celebration evening with family or friends. We both plan, because we both know we aren't skilled enough to wing it! We plan what we are going to do *up to and including* the event, and we plan what we are going to do *after* the event.

## • Planning what to do up to and including the event

As soon as you begin planning, and as you start thinking about the event, you are already making a choice to be in charge and not to drift into eating too much. Let's cover this with some chat time, including our friend Zoe.

### CHAT TIME

*ZOE: Caroline, you've always impressed me with your planning skills. Can you take us through some of your planning ideas?*

*CAROLINE: One trick I have found useful is to save up some calories in the days before the event. I eat a little less on those days, knowing that at the event, the food is going to make me want to spend some extra calories. It is up to you what you cut out or trim down on, but I bear in mind that 'low calorie-dense' foods (vegetables, salad, and lean protein) keep me fuller for longer, as well as being good for me.*

*ZOE: I understand that's useful for the days before the event, but what do you do on the day itself?*

*CAROLINE: I also eat lightly before the event itself. Then I always eat something just before the event. I think the risk of eating far too much of something like 'birthday food' is even greater if I am also genuinely hungry.*

*ZOE: I understand all of this, but isn't it difficult to juggle all of those calorie reductions and extra calories?*

*STEVE: It probably was in years gone by, but nowadays there are lots of online tools that will do that for you.*

*CAROLINE: Yes, one reason Steve and I like Nutracheck, the app that we use, is that it allows you to select one or more days a week where you will have more calories. It then works out how many calories are left for the other days – this can be a helpful tool.*

*ZOE: I understand what you are both saying, but wouldn't it be easier just to cut down afterwards, when you know how far over you have gone?*

*CAROLINE: In theory that's right, but you probably know that in the dieting game things do not always work out as the theory says it will. For instance, I tried what you are suggesting for thirty years of my life – and every time I ended up overweight!*

*STEVE: The same here, except for me it was fifty years!*

- **Planning what to do after the event**

Firstly, there may be some good news! Bodies being the mystery they often are, you might wake up on that morning after and find that you have put on little or no weight from when you started your planning.

And so you don't have to reduce calories if you don't want to. This has happened to us several times, and maybe it's not so surprising. After all, if the event was just a meal (not a two-week all-inclusive cruise!) and you saved some calories before the event and then took a little care during the event, everything might balance out. You might well end up the same weight as you were a few days before. Dieting is occasionally kind!

But it's not wise to *assume* that dieting is going to be kind. We therefore also plan what we are going to do *after* the event. This is simply a reversed version of Caroline's trick above of saving up some calories in the days before the event – now we are planning on saving some calories in the days *after* the event. What is important here is that we are planning to do it. We do not wake up the morning after going way over calories and are somehow surprised to have put on some weight. We knew this was probably going to happen (because, as you will know by now, we are both dedicated calorie counters), and we knew we were going to have to be a little careful with our calories. Now we just have to do it!

Remember that we are only talking here about putting on small amounts of weight, and so we are only talking about taking a little care – before, during, and after the event. This is not tough and drastic action. Putting on half a stone after a cruise is different, and we will look at gains like that soon.

Now, a little warning bell! We should say at this point that there are diet experts who say that deliberately eating fewer calories to compensate for an overeating event is not the right way to do it. They give good reasons for saying that increasing eating and drinking for special events is not a good idea. One of the best reasons is that some people have so many special events in their lives that they don't have enough proper 'diet days' for them to lose weight. We do understand this view, and it is certainly good if you can keep on an even pattern of calories on all days. The difficulty we see is that few people seem able to do that, and that includes us. So we think that, for most people, the 'saving calories for a bit of a blowout' is the technique that is most likely to succeed.

**Plan for a series of events**
What we have talked about so far is how to handle single over-calorie events (we gave the example of a celebration evening with family or friends). We hope you have found our thoughts useful. Unfortunately, there is something else to watch out for – when you are not trying to

handle a single over-calorie event, but instead an over-calorie weekend or an over-calorie two-week holiday!

Almost certainly you know exactly what we mean, but let's just give you an example anyway. Imagine you are one of those people who finds it difficult to lose weight. You go away for a week's holiday, come home, and find that you are half a stone heavier than when you left. It had taken you ages to lose those seven pounds! You get really fed up, think 'what's the point?' and then you give up. Of course, there are people who think, 'Oh well, it's not a real weight gain, so never mind, it will drop off again soon,' but there are not so many such serene individuals. Most people take it quite hard. So that's the problem – what's the solution?

Well, as often happens in the world of weight loss, there are no magic answers to how to lose a lot of weight gained over, say, a two-week holiday. Maybe we could follow the same sort of thinking that we have been working through above, when we looked at what to do about a single celebration. In that case we could trim our calories before (and let's use this as our example) the two-week cruise, be careful on the cruise, then trim our calories after the cruise. In principle that would work, but in real life, for most people, *we very much doubt it, and we do not recommend it.*

That may surprise you! After all, we are often suggesting in this book how to fix some dieting problem, but now we seem to be ignoring the obvious solution to a big holiday weight gain. Let us explain!

There are a few people who lose weight fairly easily. Those fortunate types include people with a high calorie burn, who have the luxury of being able to lose weight while still eating a lot. They are very much the exception.

For many people (maybe most people), the reality is that they do not have a high calorie burn, and the only way they can lose weight is to consume a modest number of calories day after day. In a nutshell, they are trying hard already. We think that it's not a good idea for those people to try to compensate for the effects of a two-week cruise by cutting down on calories before and after the cruise. The cruise will cause so much 'damage' to their diet that they will probably do one of two things: (1) cut their daily calorie intake to an unhealthy level, which is absolutely not recommended, or (2) they will persevere at a reasonable daily calorie intake, but it will take such a long time to 'undo the damage' that it will make for a miserable existence, and they may get fed up and give up.

We suggest, therefore, that if you know you have some long social event in the near future, do enjoy it, but accept that you will end up having gained some weight. That may put back the date when you hit your target weight, but that's better than jeopardising your health or giving up. In any case, you may not gain as much weight as you fear if you follow our ideas about eating on holiday (later in this slice).

One last thought in this section is that compensating for something like holiday weight gains is different once you get to maintenance. We will look at that in slice 48.

**Choose carefully what you eat at social events**

A little saying that we both find useful is 'You don't have control over what you are offered, but you always have control over what you eat.' We're not sure who first said it, but it's powerful. To put it another way, and a bit more brutally, just because you see it doesn't mean you have to eat it – you need to choose carefully what you eat. Perfect examples are the 'bring-and-share' type events and holidays, so let's have a look at those.

• **Bring-and-share eating**

'Bring-and-share' events are particularly difficult – there is an array of different foods to eat, but choosing is difficult because the array often includes a lot of fatty, high-calorie items. However, you can make sure that the array includes lower-calorie items that you are sure to enjoy – you can take some yourself! Interestingly, such low-calorie options are rarely left over. Steve would like to say at this point that Caroline is particularly good at making delicious low-calorie items, such as watermelon and feta salad or chopped-up fresh pineapple as part of a pudding. Make things like that yourself at the next bring-and-share you go to and see how popular you are!

It's important to choose carefully what you eat at bring-and-shares. Here is a blog of specific guidelines that Caroline came up with for herself:

Caroline's blog about bring-and-share eating

• I don't eat pastry at bring-and-share events. It is rarely wonderful, often soggy, and usually high-calorie. It's not worth the calories.

• I don't eat the crisps. Crisps are easily available any time I want from a shop, so why spend calories on them now?

- I avoid salads with rich and creamy dressings or that contain a lot of pasta or rice.
- I choose foods that look interesting.
- I eat a portion of anything that looks lower in calories.
- I am more likely to go for dishes that are homemade. If something is shop-bought, I can buy that version another time – there's no need to spend a lot of calories on it now.
- Unless something is totally delicious or an old favourite, I only have a single portion of anything. I (almost) never go back for seconds!
- It's helpful to drink a good amount of low-calorie drinks. Water is a great choice – it has zero calories and is almost always available.

## • Holidays

Choosing carefully what you eat on holiday is something that defeats many people – it seems so difficult that people often make little attempt to do it. Steve thinks that Caroline is unusually good at controlling calories when on holiday – so good, in fact, that most of this section is based on another of her blogs.

Caroline's blog about holiday eating

A long time ago I decided that the 'holiday calories don't count' approach didn't work for me. It undermined the habits I wanted to develop – habits of moderate and healthy eating and drinking. On the other hand, I liked food, and eating out was a part of a holiday for me. I never forgot that a diet is not a punishment! So for my next holiday, I needed a plan! But first, I needed a list of my thoughts about holidays and diets.
- Eating a lot of high-calorie food just because I am on holiday is never my best holiday memory.
- Feeling bad about my holiday because I overeat is a waste of a good holiday.
- My idea of 'eating well' on holiday is of eating out on nice, fresh, maybe unusual food – not simply eating lots of rich, sweet, creamy food (though some of that may be included).
- There are lots of things I don't stop doing just because I'm on holiday (brushing my teeth, locking the door, looking

when I cross the road, applying sun cream), so why would I stop thinking about eating healthily?

• I don't think much (or at all) about how much of my holiday eating is actually essential to the enjoyment of my holiday and how much is merely 'what I usually eat on holiday'.

That thinking resulted in my holiday plan. But – and it's a big but – this was *my* thinking and *my* plan, based on what *I* particularly like. We are all different, and we all have to problem-solve to find our own solutions. It's never a waste of your time to re-read slice 12 about learning to problem-solve!

So after all that thinking, my plan for the holiday was:

Typical holiday: have treats at the airport.
Plan: use the days travelling to and from my destination as normal diet days.

Typical holiday: pastries for breakfast, often with butter and jam.
Plan: I can easily cut out the pastries for breakfast – I can get them at home any time. I love fresh fruit and I know there will be an abundance of good-quality fruit, such as peaches, nectarines, mango, melon, and apricots. And plain yogurt is always available. So it's fruit and yogurt for breakfast!

Typical holiday: eating out once (sometimes twice) a day.
Plan: I am going self-catering and will usually only have one meal out a day. I will have salad for lunch, whether I am eating out or not. I like bread, but I don't need it every day; I'll have it only every other day, and only with lunch.

Typical holiday: cocktails, lager, or wine with both lunch and dinner.
Plan: I reckon that if I want alcohol twice a day, I will have a bigger problem than simply the need to lose weight! I plan to have sparkling water or low-alcohol lager at lunchtime.

Typical holiday: nibbles (usually crisps and nuts) and alcohol before the evening meal.

Plan: I feel that nibbles with a drink in the early evening *are* essential to my holiday pleasure. But I will make a substitution and have nibbles such as cut-up carrot and cucumber, gherkins, and silverskin onions, together with a few olives. That way I will get a nice crunch and lovely sharp tastes but far fewer calories. I will start with a glass of sparkling water, then I will have a low-alcohol lager before moving onto alcohol. Even then, I will alternate alcohol and water.

So that was how Caroline learned to plan for holidays. Anyone can learn to do it and come up with their own plan for holiday eating – still having a fantastic holiday, but saving thousands of calories at the same time!

### Enjoy what you eat

There is no point in a social eating event if you are not enjoying what you are eating! We think that there are three parts to enjoying what you are eating, as follows.

**Have food that you like on your plate.** Steve is not keen on cold sausages – he would never choose to have them at home, so he doesn't want to have them when he is out. He thinks that if he has limited calories to 'spend', then it's better to spend them on what he likes. Occasionally there is social pressure to eat foods that you don't really want to eat – we will get to that shortly.

**Concentrate on what you are eating.** Notice the flavours, textures, and scents of the food. You will probably recognise this as 'mindfulness', which we discussed in slice 19.

**Don't feel guilty because you have eaten more calories than normal.** There is only one thing sillier than carelessly overeating when you are trying to lose weight. That is carelessly overeating when you are trying to lose weight, *then* making yourself feel really bad and spoiling all the enjoyment of it! Despite everything we have said in this slice (and in the whole book, really), everyone, at some time or other, will do something that is unhelpful to their weight-loss ambitions. When we do, we should enjoy it and, in the cold light of day, just put it down to experience.

### Manage social pressures

We have covered a lot of ground in this slice about handling social eating events. But there is something that can undermine most of the techniques and advice we have talked about, and that is the social pressures you may experience when you try to apply the techniques and advice. Before we start this section, you may like to revisit slice 10, which gave a general introduction to the subject of social pressures.

Social eating is one of the trickiest challenges for a dieter to manage – many of us have too many friends and relatives for dieting to be easy! We have birthdays, weddings, celebrations, and informal get-togethers, usually involving food and alcohol. These enjoyable events can be socially awkward for a dieter to negotiate.

Steve has handled these difficult social moments in a pretty robust way, just telling people that he was on a strict diet. And if he was presented with calorific food, he (1) had a small portion or (2) ate just the parts that were not too calorific (he remembers picking out pieces of salmon from a salmon en croute, leaving all the delicious pastry on his plate) or (3) just didn't touch it at all. He thinks that he did upset a couple of people, but everyone else just accepted it.

Many might find Steve's approach too tough; people usually want to keep all of their friends! Caroline may be more socially skilled than Steve, and so we are going to look at the sort of approach Caroline favours. Let's look at a little more chat time.

### CHAT TIME

*ZOE: My problem is simply that my social life gets in the way of losing weight! I can do quite well with watching what I eat on an ordinary working day, but the problem comes when my partner and I want to eat out. Or we have a meal with friends at their house and they serve food that is high-calorie. Or even just when my daughter comes home for the weekend and I don't want to offer her salad and diet food.*

*CAROLINE: I know exactly what you mean, and sometimes I think managing my weight would be easier if I had no friends, no family, no social events, nothing ever to celebrate, and there were no interesting places to eat out! However, I am a very lucky woman because I do have all of these 'problems'!*

*ZOE: But I know that you are a successful dieter and maintainer, so how do you handle these social problems? I see that things are difficult, but not impossible, for an event you've planned for and maybe brought some food to. But what about a spontaneous event when there is little choice – how do you handle that without causing offence?*

CAROLINE: Ah, yes, that's what I call a tartiflette moment.

ZOE: A what?!

CAROLINE: I had a completely unexpected invitation to dinner with some friends for that same evening. I was fairly near the start of my diet, and I was being particularly careful. I hadn't saved calories during the week, it was obviously not a 'bring-and-share' type of event, and I had no idea what would be served.

ZOE: What did you do?

CAROLINE: I went, delighted to have been invited by a fairly new friend and thinking, 'Well, I'll try and make wise choices about what I eat.'

ZOE: What happened?

CAROLINE: The hostess put two dishes on the table. One was a smallish bowl of salad. The other was an enormous dish of tartiflette. It smelled delicious and I asked what was in it. The answer was: potatoes, butter, bacon lardons, white wine, onions, cream, and a lot of cheese. I immediately realised that it was going to blow my diet out of the water. This was confirmed when I estimated the calories on the following day – a portion ranged between 850 and 1,200 calories.

ZOE: What did you do?

CAROLINE: I ate it. I had a normal-sized portion, the same as everyone else (though I didn't have the garlic bread on offer as well!). I didn't feel guilty about it. I just enjoyed it – in fact, I loved it.

ZOE: I know that you are a big fan of getting on the scales – I suppose that you checked to see if that meal stopped your weight loss.

CAROLINE: Yes! I weighed myself the next morning and found that my weight had gone up a little. But I immediately addressed the problem – on that next day I was particularly *strict. I had porridge for breakfast, salad and prawns (no dressing) for lunch, and stir-fry and chicken for dinner (no rice, but masses of vegetables, 'fried' with only two sprays of oil). The result was that my small weight gain had disappeared.*

We think that the important message here is that you can plan particularly carefully, but sooner or later you will be in a situation where refusing to eat something that is very calorific without giving offence is extremely difficult. Or simply that the food is so desirable to you that you just want to eat it, regardless of the calories.

In such situations, we think there is a good case to just eat it and enjoy it without guilt (see above!). Our opinion is that there are just two things to be concerned about:

• Being so worried by any sudden weight gain that you get fed up and give up. We covered that earlier in this slice.

• Falling into the trap of doing it often. This is an easy trap to fall into because if you 'just eat it' once, it makes it easier to do it again and again. In the end, you 'just eat it' so often that you are not really dieting at all. In which case, you may need to have another read of slice 3.

# Slice 23

# Increase your calories burned

We have already said (especially in slice 9) that it's more important to control calories consumed than calories burned. You may remember that nearly everyone who loses or maintains weight does so mainly thanks to controlling what they consume; controlling what they burn by exercising is less important. It is a rare and athletic person who achieves their weight goals mostly by exercising, with just a little help from watching what they eat and drink. Because we believe this so firmly, we have concentrated so far in this book on looking at what we consume.

We do need to make ourselves clear, though. There is nothing at all wrong with doing exercise – working out in a gym, pounding the streets training for long-distance runs, vigorous swimming, etc. This will help weight loss no end. But what we worry about – and we have seen it happen often – is when people who want to lose weight believe the story that exercise is the key to all weight loss. For whatever reason, they can't or don't want to exercise, so they are immediately discouraged and feel that their dieting efforts are doomed to failure. That is simply not true – weight loss is perfectly possible without doing any exercise at all.

But yes, burning more calories is good, and we will now look at how you can increase your calories burned. We are going to be talking here about physical exercise. You do read from time to time about how more calories can be burned by other means, such as eating certain foodstuffs, drinking cold water, or even thinking hard. But we have not seen any convincing, authoritative evidence that these work to any significant extent. Physical exercise definitely *does* work, so that is what we are going to concentrate on.

## Starting to do exercise

When many people think about starting to do exercise, they have a self-defeating thought (you may remember those from slice 5). The thought is 'I've never exercised and I can't now.' They have never got into the habit of exercising, and they just don't see themselves as an exercise sort of person. Both of us had similar self-defeating thoughts, so let's have some chat time.

## CHAT TIME

*STEVE: I was quite surprised to hear that you were a non-exerciser, because you are someone who is always looking for an opportunity to walk.*

*CAROLINE: That's true – now. But although I was mildly sporty when I was young, once I left the organised sport of school, I didn't really move much at all, and I didn't want to, either. Looking back on it now, I was a bit of a sloth!*

*STEVE: What was it that converted a sloth into a gazelle?*

*CAROLINE: An interesting one. It was basically an article I read – that most successful weight-maintainers control calories consumed and they also exercise (often 10,000 steps a day). That's when I realised that I had no real way of measuring my exercise, so I bought a cheap pedometer.*

*STEVE: Did that confirm what you thought about your lack of exercise?*

*CAROLINE: Yes! It told me that I usually struggled to do 2,500 steps a day. That spurred me on to find some nice places to walk, and as I lost weight, walking became easier. I became fitter, I walked more, and I lost weight. And so on. It was a really pleasurable 'virtuous circle'! What about you?*

*STEVE: In my youth, I was bulky but modestly sporty. I was still pretty active into my forties, but I think my increasing weight began to slow me down and made exercising much less fun. Then I had a leg injury, which I didn't properly recover from, and that was it – I became a sloth too. Some years later, my knees started to hurt, and then I was convinced that my exercise days were completely over.*

*CAROLINE: It seems funny because ever since I've known you, you never have a pair of trainers and a rucksack far away, and most of your holidays include a lot of walking. How did you break away from being a sloth?*

*STEVE: I saw a physiotherapist about my knee pain, and she said that the best thing I could do was lose some weight and that exercise would help me to achieve that. I had that old self-defeating thought that I couldn't do any exercise because of my knees.*

*CAROLINE: Sounds like an excuse to me!*

*STEVE: I think that's what she thought too. She asked me how far I could walk, and I said about thirty steps, so she said OK, do that, and tomorrow do thirty-five steps. I did, and so it went on. A few weeks later, I was counting steps in the hundreds, and then in the thousands. And after a year I was averaging the magic 10,000 steps a day myself.*

The message from this chat is that some sort of exercise is usually possible. You might need to start with limited exercise, but if you keep trying, most people can work their way up to a useful number of calories burned. And it's more than that – walking is healthy, enjoyable, and fun!

There is another self-defeating thought we hear a lot of, and that is that people haven't got a gym nearby or can't afford to join one or don't want to show their big bodies in front of various toned gods and goddesses and, therefore, they cannot do any exercise. We cannot say it strongly enough – you do *not* need to go to a gym to burn calories!

There is nothing wrong with gyms, but simple walking is an excellent form of exercise because it needs no particular skills and it is cheap. It also gets you out in the fresh air, which makes you feel good! OK, OK, if the weather is really bad, you might not want to go out, but in that case you can walk inside your house. OK, OK, your house is too small, but in that case there are plenty of videos that you can watch and walk along to, more or less on the spot. No more excuses – just use those problem-solving skills we told you all about (slice 12)!

**Keeping going with exercise**
So you have brushed aside any self-defeating thoughts and you have taken the first step (literally) to exercise, whether it is in some high-tech gym or walking in the open air. The question now is how to keep going. It's quite hard to take that first step, but it's even harder to be still exercising a month later.

Your lifestyle has a strong influence on your ability to exercise. Not just the time it takes but also the flexibility it requires of your life –

for example, most people we know who are exercise fiends do not have full-time jobs. It's fitting exercise into your life that gives rise to another self-defeating thought: 'I don't have time to exercise.' This is the difficult bit, and where it is hard for anyone to help you. Exercise is a really good idea, but it certainly needs time, and you have to figure out how you are going to carve out that time in your life. And that is a task that may be impossible if you try to carve out time for something you don't enjoy. If you find something you really enjoy doing, the time you need to do it often miraculously appears!

So we think the key to finding time to exercise is finding which exercise you really like. It might be training in a gym, it might be (like us) walking in the country, or it might be any one of a thousand other possibilities. We met someone who had never raised a sweat in their lives, but then they had a go at a very slow jog and a year later they were training for a marathon. And another who was in her fifties, could not swim, had some lessons at the local pool, loved it, and is now an open-water swimmer. There is an activity out there with your name on it. You just need to find it!

But whatever you decide to do, we would urge you to measure it. If, for example, your 'thing' is going to be walking, then get yourself a pedometer. If you want to, you could get some wearable device that costs a lot of money, measures all sorts of stuff, and that you are proud to display on your arm (until it goes out of fashion, of course). But a simple pedometer costs next to nothing and does the basics – in other words, it counts your steps. Guess what we both use, given that we both have a keen eye on value for money!

And don't worry about the accuracy of whatever device you choose. You are trying to increase your exercise, and if, for example, you are walking, what is important is to keep doing it and try to keep increasing it a little. It doesn't matter whether you are walking 8,460 steps in a day or 8,218.

So measuring your exercise is good, but recording it is even better. On a phone or on a scrap of paper? Again, that's not important. What matters is recording it somewhere, because then you can see how your amount of exercise has changed over time. It is motivating to see your exercise numbers going up and up. On the other hand, it is also useful to show that your exercise numbers are going down when you could have sworn that they were going up!

Measuring also gives you the ability – if you are numbers inclined – to come up with some fun and motivating thoughts. For example:

• Steve recorded his steps for a whole year and saw that he had taken over three and a half million steps – 1,200 miles.
• The steps that Caroline took in one year worked off two stone.

**Exercise SPCs (Small Permanent Changes)**
We have already discussed (in slice 13) how weight-loss success is increased by making small permanent changes (SPCs) to what you eat and drink, as well as always being on the lookout for *new* small permanent changes. The good news is that weight-loss success is also increased by making small permanent changes (SPCs) to calories burned.

As with SPCs to calories consumed, the challenge with SPCs to calories burned is figuring out which SPCs are going to work in your own particular case. Unless you are deeply committed to a full-on exercise regime (and you have the available time to follow such a regime), you may find that the best SPCs are quite modest – changes that are going to be easy to adopt for a long time, maybe forever.

These are all nice words, but let us give you some exercise SPCs that have worked for us. We'll also show which of us they apply to, illustrating how people are different and how we all have to figure out what works for each of us (that problem-solving idea yet again).
• Get off the bus a stop before the one you really want (applies to Caroline; Steve doesn't use buses).
• Park the car at the far end of the supermarket car park (applies to both Caroline and Steve).
• Walk the long way round to the garden shed (applies to Steve, because he does a lot of his work in a garden shed, so he never goes to the shed by the quickest route but walks around the garden first!).
• Don't use lifts (applies to both Caroline and Steve, although they both break this 'rule' in certain circumstances – for example, if they need to go to the 27th floor!).
• Walk to shops you previously would have driven to (applies to both Caroline and Steve).
• Go swimming much more (applies to Caroline; Steve is not keen on swimming).

If you are not sure whether a change is worth making, have a rough guess at the calories you will save in a year – remember every 3,500 calories is a pound off. This will make it much more real to you. For example, Steve's little detour to get to his garden shed works off an extra four pounds in a year. It's a trivial change, which he hardly notices, but just that little bit of additional activity burns off nearly a stone in three years!

And one final thought about the benefit to your diet of exercise – while you are exercising, whether it's pumping iron, swimming, running, or just wandering down to the garden shed, you are much less likely to be *eating* anything!

# Slice 24

# Weigh yourself regularly and record it

If your target is to lose weight, you will only know for sure that you are going in the right direction if you weigh yourself!

Even if your target is not to get to a certain weight but rather to fit into a certain size of clothes, weighing can still be useful along the way. If you want to know whether the way you are trying to slim down is working, the scales will tell you much more quickly than the feel of your clothes. After all, even half a stone may not make a huge difference to the way most of your clothes fit. And a gain of half a stone, without knowing it, is not good news. So please read the rest of this slice, even if you are not yet convinced about the value of weighing yourself!

If you are already weighing yourself regularly (somewhere between once a day and once a week) and you are recording those weighings, then you can probably skip this slice. But before you turn to the next one, you might like to know that you already have something in common with many successful long-term maintainers. That's because research tells us that most of those people weigh that often.

The rest of this slice answers five important questions dieters often ask about weighing:

## Why is it important to weigh regularly?
Weighing regularly is important because information is power! Knowing whether your weight is going up, down, or staying the same will enable you to keep track of whether your diet strategy is working for you. If it isn't working, then – assuming you are someone who takes weight management seriously (surely you are!) – you'll want to change the way you are dieting.

There is a bonus. If you are losing weight and keeping close track of it by weighing regularly, the tracking becomes motivating in itself. It helps you to keep going and to continue making good food choices. Equally, a weight that is going in the wrong direction can motivate you to look at what you have been eating and see if there are changes you need to make.

And there is another bonus! Weighing regularly is a message to yourself that you are someone who is taking dieting seriously. The message is even stronger when you record your weight in such a way that you can keep track of it over the long term. When being 'someone who is taking dieting seriously' becomes part of how you see yourself, making good food choices will be easier. That is because humans get an uncomfortable feeling when what they think and what they actually do contradict each other. People then want to change either what they think or what they do in order to feel better.

In dieting terms, people often feel bad or guilty when they have a calorie allowance for the day but eat something that takes them over that allowance (let's say chocolate cake). They can make themselves feel better either by

**changing what they think** by saying to themselves, 'Oh well, it's a special occasion and I don't need to diet on special occasions' and **sticking to what they do** by eating the chocolate cake
OR
**sticking to what they think** by saying, 'I want a piece of chocolate cake, but I won't have it, because I intend to come within my calorie allowance today and that would take me over' and **changing what they do** by *not* eating the chocolate cake.

Whichever they decide to do, people feel better – because what they think and what they do are in line with one another. But obviously for a dieter, the better choice is the second – because the chocolate cake is not eaten! And regularly weighing makes it more likely that they will choose that second one because they see themselves as a dieter, and so more likely to make that diet-friendly second choice.

Having in mind all those good reasons for weighing regularly and keeping a record of your weight (so you can see how it changes), let's look at some other common questions.

### How often should I weigh myself?

Somewhere between once a day and once a week seems to be ideal. As we said above, something that many long-term maintainers have in common is that they weigh themselves with that regularity.

It's important to bear in mind, whether you weigh daily or weekly, that your weight may be a 'blip' – body weight can fluctuate for what seems to be no reason. When the blip is a blip upwards, many people get discouraged (they are absolutely fine when it's a blip downwards!).

We both weigh daily, record those weights, and later work out the average weight for the week (some apps do that for you). We like this average weight system because it smooths out those discouraging day-to-day blips. But we freely admit that we like playing with numbers, so it's not for everyone!

Weekly weighers do sometimes have a look at their weight more often than weekly, and that's not a problem. But we do have some concern when we hear people call these extra weighings 'cheating', 'being naughty', or 'having a sneaky peak'. Dieting is hard enough as it is, without giving yourself something more to get cross about! But it's your body (and probably your scales), so weigh yourself whenever it suits you. Whenever you do weigh yourself, however, we recommend that you record it. Read on!

**Do I really have to record every single weight?**
A lot of people get discouraged if they step on the scales and find that their weight has gone up. They sometimes deal with this by recording *only the losses*. If you record only the weights that you like the look of, there is the danger of your weight drifting upwards without you realising that's what is happening. It is the recording and paying attention to the upward drift that is so helpful in pushing you to think about what you are doing (or not doing).

Weighing regularly *and recording* (1) gives you that message that you are serious about dieting, (2) helps you not to fool yourself, and (3) gives you a prod to review your eating and drinking if your weight is going in the wrong direction. Not recording undermines all of these things that help keep you motivated. So we think that recording your weighings is a good idea. Recording also becomes encouraging and motivating in itself. And (another one for number-lovers here) having a curve on a graph that is heading downwards is a huge added incentive to keep going!

**What do changes in my weight really mean?**
What is most important to get right *before* you step on the scales is to understand what today's weight really means.

First, let's think about what it does **not** mean. Your weight is **not** a measure of your worth, your value, or how lovable you are. Your weight is **not** a measure of your character. Having lost weight since you weighed previously (whenever that was) does **not** make you a better person, **nor** one with more willpower. Not having lost weight when you expected does **not** make you a worse or a weaker person. Any one weight is **not** a measure of how successful a dieter you are, and it does **not** predict whether you will be able to lose weight in the long term. Your weight today will **not** predict the way the day goes or the health and happiness of the people you love. In fact, in terms of everything that really matters, your weight today is utterly unimportant!

But we have just said that weight *is* important! True, so what *does* your weight mean? It is an extremely useful piece of information about how much you weigh today. It tells you, broadly speaking, whether what you are doing to lose weight is working for you or whether, sooner or later, you might need to tweak what you are doing.

Your weight is, however, a difficult friend to read! It takes into account many factors, including:

• **What you have eaten and drunk in the past few hours.** If you have drunk a couple of pints of any liquid – water, beer, tea, fruit juice, soup, or a combination of them all – and you have not been to the bathroom in the last couple of hours, you will weigh a couple of pounds more than you did before you drank them. Liquid is heavy stuff!

If you have eaten a meal in the last few hours, the food will be in your system still and, whatever it weighed when you put it on the plate, it will still weigh inside you. It may therefore be best to weigh yourself in the morning, before you have had anything to eat or drink and after getting rid of both types of your body waste matter (you know what we mean!).

If you work nights, it all gets more complicated, but perhaps weighing after your long daytime sleep would be the best alternative.

• **What you have eaten and drunk in the past few days.** As examples: (1) When your body stores carbohydrates it also stores water, so suddenly eating more carbohydrates will make most people temporarily put on even more weight in the form of water. But it's not weight caused by extra fat. (2) If you have had some meat-heavy meals, the meat can be slower for your body to digest, and so it will 'sit around' in your system for a while. (3) If you have eaten a lot of salt, you may find (like many people) that you weigh more because of retained water.

• If you are a woman, **hormones will play a part** – a bigger part for some women than for others. A rise in weight because of fluid retention just before your period is not unusual.

• If you are **constipated**, which can happen for all sorts of different reasons, this will up your weight a little.

• **Scales vary and batteries run down**, so use the same scales, always put them in the same place, and change the batteries often.

• **Clothes and shoes do not all weigh the same**, so wear the same weight of clothes. Weighing naked works well, although you may not want to do this if you weigh yourself in Boots or some other public place!

All the above means that your weight on any given day is just a snapshot of what is happening to your weight. It is 'true' but not the whole truth. However, if you are keeping to your calorie allowance and keeping a record of your weighings over a reasonable period of time, then you will see that you are losing weight. Even if your weight is up one day because of something on the above list, the trend will be downwards. And if you have a good record of how things are going over the longer term, you will be less likely to get fed up and give up.

**I just really hate weighing myself – do I have to?**
Some people may understand everything we have written in this slice, but they just hate weighing themselves. If that sounds like you, here are two possible alternative approaches to regular weighing.

The first approach is simply *not* to weigh yourself. This approach can work, but it can take a long time to see whether your dieting is succeeding or whether it is going off track. And it is also a high-risk approach because if you finally *do* weigh yourself and find that you have not lost much, you may get fed up and give up.

The second approach is not to weigh yourself, but *instead* take body measurements or note your dress size (or male equivalent). This approach can work well if you have a lot of weight to lose because (1) people who are very overweight often do not like scales, especially not if they have to use them in a public place, or (2) you cannot find scales that measure such a high weight (Steve was in that situation for many years).

While we believe that neither of the above approaches is as reliable as weighing yourself, they can nevertheless be motivating and are better than nothing. Especially if you actually record any measurements you do take (see earlier in this slice for the benefits of recording measurements).

# Slice 25

# Don't be discouraged if you haven't lost as much as you 'should have'

You have tried so hard to lose weight. You have made sacrifices. You have not eaten as much as you wanted of what you love to eat. You may have taken exercise for the first time in many a long year. Now all you need is a little encouragement when you step on the scales.

You are being realistic. You have fully taken on board what we said in the previous slice, that weight can fluctuate for any number of reasons in the short term – so you have left it a reasonable time since your last weighing. You have also calculated roughly how much weight you should have lost.

The moment has arrived. You step on the scales, and they tell you that you have lost nowhere near as much as you should have, or maybe you haven't lost anything, or maybe – incredible but true – you have actually gained weight!

It is at that point that an awful lot of people get fed up and give up. And that point can come a week after the diet started, a month after, or three years after. Any time is a good time to give up in the face of the horrible unfairness of dieting hard and failing to lose the weight *you should have lost*.

Even worse is that if you soldier on, the failure to lose what you should have lost can continue for weeks or even months. And in that case, it is often referred to as a diet plateau. Being on a diet plateau is particularly frustrating and a common reason to give up a diet. We can help you through this problem, but we do need to look at what is going on here. There seems to be a lot of unfairness involved.

The root of a feeling of unfairness may be that you have an idea of roughly how much you 'should have lost'. We all have a lot of knowledge nowadays, thanks to apps that count our calories consumed and apps that tell us how many calories we burn. And many of us know that a pound of body fat equals about 3,500 calories. So we put these together, and that gives us an expectation of what we should be losing. We know roughly what the result should be for all the effort we put in.

The difficulty is that our idea of how much we should have lost is based on calorie deficit, although we may not use those words. In slice 6 we introduced the term 'calorie deficit', meaning the situation where

you consume fewer calories than your body needs. So your idea of the weight you should have lost is only going to be reasonable if you know
• the calories in everything you eat and drink,
• the calories your body needs for the exercise you take, and
• the calories your body needs simply to keep you alive.
Let's look at each of these in turn.

### The calories in everything you eat and drink
If you are following a calorie-counting diet, it is easy to get a reasonable idea of how many calories you are eating and drinking. We have already seen that there are plenty of websites that give you the information that you need. But there are two possible problems:

**You may not be recording everything you have consumed.** Maybe you were rather fed up with strict calorie counting, and you really, really wanted to eat or drink something, but it would have put you over your calorie allowance, so you had what you wanted but didn't record it. Your idea of what weight you should have lost was hence too optimistic because of the chocolate cake you forgot about.

People often get annoyed when it is suggested that they have failed to record something they have eaten or drunk, and maybe you have never done it yourself. But the fact is that research has shown time and time again that a large proportion of people do seriously under-record their calories consumed.

**Your recording of calories consumed may be lower than it should have been because of 'weight control fatigue'.** Weight control fatigue is when our diet activities slip over time; for example, if you have begun to estimate calories rather than use the kitchen scales. This is perfectly understandable, but you need to be careful.

Steve's experience of weight control fatigue started with carefully weighing out 40 grams of porridge oats every morning – that's 150 calories. But a couple of years later, he had drifted away from proper weighing of food. He wanted to accelerate his weight loss but was having trouble doing it – so he went back to basics by weighing absolutely everything. He found that his normal portion had become 60 grams – that's 225 calories. A good example of weight control fatigue.

OK, 75 calories may not be the end of the world. But if you have weight control fatigue that affects several items every day, it probably makes the difference between a good weight loss and putting weight on. So our advice is to keep up-to-date with exactly what you are consuming, and that will keep weight control fatigue at bay, and *that* will help your idea of your calorie deficit to be realistic.

**The calories your body needs for the exercise you take**

If you are recording everything you consume and you are managing to avoid weight control fatigue, then, as we said above, you should be able to have a good idea of your calories consumed. *But that is not the case with your calories burned.* In fact, unless you are exercising in a laboratory, any estimate you make of calories burned is probably inaccurate.

As a single example, we have just consulted a website to find out the calories burned when walking. The site shows that an hour of walking on the flat at 2 mph burns 150 calories, walking at 4 mph burns 320 calories, and walking upstairs burns 590 calories. But if you walked for an hour, would you really know at what speed you were walking? Was some of it uphill or downhill? Did you stop for a short rest (especially walking upstairs)? And those figures are the same for women and men, for all ages, for all levels of fitness, and for all body weights.

In other words – again, except for a scientific study – the calorific value of your hour of walking can only be a broad approximation of what you actually burned, whatever source you used to get the information. And that applies to every form of exercise you might take.

The danger is that you do some exercise, maybe overestimate the intensity of the exercise, and maybe use the figures for calories burned from a source that's on the high side. That will then show you a calorie deficit that is higher than the one you really created. And there is a further danger – having overestimated your exercise calories, you then eat more, wrongly thinking that you have 'earned' those additional calories. So, all in all, it is a good idea to be particularly cautious and conservative when you measure your exercise calories.

**The calories your body needs simply to keep you alive**

We have now seen in this slice that there are real difficulties in knowing the calories in what we eat and drink and – even more – in knowing the calories we burn when exercising. But even if we could know both of those things reasonably accurately, we would still have enormous difficulty in knowing how much weight we 'should' lose. And that is because incredible complexities are taking place in our bodies under the heading of 'metabolism' (the processes in our bodies that keep us alive and our organs working properly). Our metabolism is difficult to quantify in terms of calories, but it can change for many different reasons, such as age or illness.

It is possible that the diet plateau we mentioned earlier happens because of our metabolism. But although an awful lot has been written on the internet linking diet plateaus and metabolism, there is no conclusive hard science on the subject. We both regard the NHS website as the 'gold standard' opinion on such matters, but, at the time of writing, that website says nothing about the reasons for diet plateaus. And it has few, if any, certainties about the link between dieting and metabolism. Interestingly, however, the site does say, 'People who struggle to lose weight often blame a slow metabolism. But there's little evidence to support this claim.'

### In conclusion
We can be sure that, over time, calorie deficits will all have exactly the effect that they should on your body weight. **They must do.** If you are not feeding your body the calories it needs to keep you alive and to do the exercise you are putting it through, it has to get the energy from somewhere, and it gets it – at some time or another – from your stores of fat.

But the big snag is the phrase 'at some time or another', because it is impossible to be accurate about when particular calorie deficits end up changing your body weight. You may have to wait a long time for your hard-earned calorie deficits to reflect in the display on your scales – perhaps until a mysterious diet plateau has passed. The risk is that you might get fed up and give up.

It's annoying. But there are two keys to getting through a period, such as a diet plateau, when you have not lost the weight you 'should have lost'. The first key is to understand why these annoyances happen, and we hope this slice has helped with that. The second key is to remember that – at some time or another – any real calorie deficits **must**, as a biological certainty, show up on the scales.

# Slice 26

# What to do to get back
# on track after straying

If you are reading this book like a novel – from start to finish – then you have now read about 60,000 words of our thoughts and advice about how to lose weight. We hope that you have found these words useful and that they have been helpful on your journey towards your target weight. But it would be silly for us to imagine that everyone's journey progresses smoothly. Many (probably most) people falter somewhere along the way, and so this slice looks at what to do if it all goes wrong.

This slice is divided into three sections:

• At what point is it right to say that you have strayed?
• How did that straying happen?
• How do you get back on track?

If you want a quick solution, you may be tempted to jump straight to the third section. But we recommend that you first read the other sections. As in many other parts of our book, we think the most benefit will come from clearly understanding the problem before grabbing a solution.

**At what point is it right to say that you have strayed?**
We see straying from your diet as meaning when weight gains become so frequent that the trend of your weight – over several weeks – is flat or is actually increasing.

To be clear, for the purposes of our book, we do not count short-term fluctuations as 'straying'. Specifically:
• We saw in slice 24 that you may weigh more on one day than on the previous day simply because of the complicated way that the human body works. This is short term and not what we mean by straying from your diet.
• Many people will exceed their calorie allowance on one day and the following day will see a genuine increase in weight. They may react badly to this. They may feel that their diet is failing and do something unwise, such as hardly eat at all or get fed up and give up. Both of these are highly undesirable – it is better to accept that you did exceed your calorie allowance and say to yourself that you should 'draw a line,

because tomorrow is another day' or something similar. But this is also short term and, again, is not what we mean by straying from your diet.

## How did that straying happen?

When you have clearly strayed, the reason for it could be one or more unhelpful-to-your-diet things that you have begun to do. It is important to have a good idea of what these unhelpful-to-your-diet things are, because knowing where you went wrong will (1) give you a good idea of what you need to do to correct the situation and (2) help you to avoid doing the same next time.

The more detailed your knowledge about the unhelpful-to-your-diet things that caused your problem, the easier it will be to get back on track. For example, if your body weight is obviously on the way up but you tell yourself it was because 'it just didn't work out this time', then that is too vague to give you guidance on what to do now or in the future if things go wrong again. So we thought that we would bare our souls and give you an idea of how we strayed from our own diets over the years.

### *CHAT TIME*

*CAROLINE: I have always had (and still have) a sweet tooth, and sometimes it has got the better of me. I have been known to eat something sweet while knowing that it would take me over my calorie allowance for the day. That is not so important once, but if life is stressful for weeks on end, then that is how straying can happen. You're not much interested in sweet foods, are you?*

*STEVE: No, but my weakness is cheese, and I have found that in the evening it has sometimes been an unsuccessful struggle to avoid going to the freezer (where we store it to stop me grabbing it), defrosting it, and having a nice big piece with an equally nice big glass of port.*

*CAROLINE: But was it all calorie counted?*

*STEVE: If only! No, by that time in the evening, calorie counting was not high on my to-do list. And, worse, once I got into the cheese habit, my diet started to stray as well. It didn't help by telling myself to draw a line and it would be OK tomorrow.*

148

*CAROLINE: Ah yes, this is the flaw in the 'draw a line' approach – if you follow that approach a lot, you may go over your allowed calories so often that you stop losing weight, and so you are no longer really 'on a diet' at all.*

*STEVE: Are there any other big issues that have led you into diet straying? I know you have often told me that it's important to think about dieting matters in the right way.*

*CAROLINE: Yes – you have been listening! Two examples of that are (1) I keep the benefits of maintaining my weight loss at the forefront of my mind by writing them down and reading them regularly and (2) I keep at bay self-defeating thoughts, such as 'I'm no good at dieting, I'll never lose all the weight I need to, so I might as well give up.' Unfortunately, I have found in the past that my success at keeping these thoughts in my mind has varied, and sometimes I have ended up straying from my diet.*

*STEVE: It's a never-ending battle.*

These are some of our experiences of what goes wrong and contributes to the straying from our own diets. One of the most important themes in the book is that we are all different and we all have to problem-solve to find our own solutions. That means that although in our chat time you might have recognised some problems that you have experienced yourself, much more important is to be clear about which problems caused *your* straying. Don't underestimate the difficulty of doing that! It needs a lot of honesty, and it is quite painful at times. We found it difficult to have that chat time ourselves, and these were problems that we experienced years ago and have (largely) overcome – but we still felt a little foolish telling you about them now.

### How do you get back on track?
This is when the honesty about what went wrong pays off! We suggest that, armed with your knowledge of *why* you strayed, you can find the slices in the book that are relevant to that problem. You can do that by simply referring to the slice titles.

Here are two examples:

**Example 1.** Perhaps you realise that the reason you strayed from your diet was because work became difficult and you found comfort in eating just what you wanted to eat. That is the ground covered by slices 4 and 20, concerning emotional eating.

**Example 2.** You may realise that your weight has increased gradually because your grandfather came to live with you and insisted on 'proper food' and not 'rabbit food'. That difficulty is the social problem of sticking to your own diet when somebody near to you wants something else. That type of situation is discussed in slices 10 and 22.

But you need to be resourceful! It would be impossible to write a book where every possible dieting problem that anyone might ever have experienced is discussed and solved. But our book does cover a lot of ground, and it has to be up to you to find the relevant sections and apply what we have written that's relevant to your own particular situation (it's problem-solving again).

On the same theme of everyone having to problem-solve to find their own solutions, we are now going to look at some chat time about solutions we arrived at ourselves. We found these particularly helpful and hope you do too.

### CHAT TIME

*STEVE: What would you say was your single most useful idea for getting back on track?*

*CAROLINE: I think mine was to go back to what I did at the start of my diet and write out a list of reasons why I wanted to lose weight, and then read that list – often!*

*STEVE: That was Judith Beck's idea, which we mentioned back in slice 3.*

*CAROLINE: Indeed. What was your most useful back-on-track idea?*

*STEVE: Mine was to go back to weighing everything I consumed and recording it in a food diary, so I could make sure that my calories were always low enough to create a calorie deficit.*

*CAROLINE: Then there was another idea that I think we both thought was important. That was going back to planning what I was going to eat for the following few days, and then only eating what I had planned!*

*STEVE: Oh yes, that's good. And there was a sort of variation on that one, where the planning was even more focused than 'the following few days' – the idea was simply to commit to dieting for a single day.*

*CAROLINE: That 'One-Day Diet' worked well for me and for many people I know. The attraction was that if the total amount of weight I needed to lose was overwhelming, or if my life was simply going through a difficult patch, then all I had to do was eat within my calorie allowance for one day. Anybody can do that! Then maybe I could do it again the next day, and the next. Then I might find myself back on track (and I often did).*

*STEVE: And another idea I know that we both rated highly was to weigh ourselves every day. It meant we got a good feeling of watching as our weight started to drop again, which encouraged us to continue.*

*CAROLINE: I have heard people say they are not going to weigh themselves again until they are back on track, because weighing themselves when they are not on track is too depressing. But that would have been disastrous on one occasion when my weight continued to increase.*

*STEVE: Of course, none of these was something to be particularly proud about – they were all examples of what we had done, let slip, then started to do again in order to get back on track.*

*CAROLINE: True, but there was something I did that was a new idea – I decided to tell somebody what was going on in my dieting life. That was the time that I gained a diet coach called Steve Marshall!*

We think that the system we have described in this slice – figuring out how your straying from the diet happened, and then going back to good ways in order to get back on track – is a good one. However, a lot of people don't have anything in particular they can put their finger on as the cause of their diets breaking down. They tend to say things as such as:
'I lost interest in the whole dieting business.'

'I just couldn't be bothered anymore.'
'Life got in the way.'
'I lost my mojo.'
'My weight is probably OK after all.'

If you feel that you could have said one of these (or similar) yourself and you are happy to stop trying to diet, then of course you should stop. If you ever change your mind, you can always start again, and our book will still be here to help you. **However**, our experience is that people who say such things do not always mean them – they can simply mean that they still want to lose weight but are finding it hard to articulate what is wrong, and they are fed up with the whole situation. If that applies to you, please read on.

We think that the most likely way of successfully restarting a diet where your interest in the subject seems to have disappeared is to go right back to basics. And the most important matter to address is your motivation to lose weight. Without motivation, nothing will happen. We suggest, therefore, that you go back to slice 3 and read it again, slowly and carefully. If you never read it in the first place, maybe thinking that you just wanted to get straight down to dieting action, then please read it particularly carefully! Slice 3 may just be what you need to ignite your enthusiasm. It will help you to see what will be so beneficial to you in being an appropriate weight.

If slice 3 is useful to you (either again or for the first time), you could also go right back to basics and re-read the whole of the book up to this point. Re-reading up to here will take you something like five hours. But, with any luck, once you have done that, you will find that this time you can get to your target weight and be ready to move on to slice 27. That slice is the beginning of part 3 of the book about how to keep at your target weight forever – an exciting moment in any dieter's journey!

But here's just a final thought in part 2. You may not be a perfect dieter, but it will stand you in very good stead indeed if you are good at quickly getting back on track.

## The Weight Maintenance Manual
### how to achieve and maintain
### your ideal weight

The four parts of The Weight Maintenance Manual are:

Part 1: What you need to understand
so you can lose weight successfully

Part 2: The actions that you need to take
so you can reach your target weight

Part 3: What you need to understand
so you can maintain your target weight forever

Part 4: The actions that you need to take
so you can maintain your target weight forever

# Welcome to

# Part 3

## What you need
## to understand
## so you can maintain your
## target weight forever

# Slice 27

# Understand why the maintenance of your weight loss is so difficult

## Reaching your target weight is a wonderful feeling of triumph!

## If you have got there ...

## HUGE CONGRATULATIONS!!!

We don't want to spoil your special moment but, unfortunately, the maintenance of your excellent weight loss may be a tricky business. In fact, many maintainers say that maintenance is harder than losing the weight in the first place.

The evidence is that most people who lose weight put it all back on again, and they often put on even more than they just lost. Certainly, we were both delighted to arrive at our target weight but also anxious about what the future might hold. But we have been largely successful with our own weight maintenance, and that is the whole reason we wrote this book – so we could help others to achieve the same.

As usual, we believe that the more you understand why something is difficult, the better placed you are to manage the difficulties. So let's begin part 3 of the book by looking at *why* maintenance of weight loss can be difficult. There are four main reasons, which we discuss in the rest of this slice.

### You were too late starting to lay down the basis for maintaining
What a strange statement! But the key to understanding it lies in what we wrote way back in slice 2 – it was about new habits. Whether or not you have been following our advice from the beginning of the book, we suggest it would be a good idea to have a look at slice 2 now. But we'll give you the headlines, which are that it's of great importance (1) to start acquiring new habits as soon as you begin your weight-loss diet, (2) to decide, deep down, that that is just the beginning of those habits, and (3) to decide that you will change very little as you reach target weight and continue into the rest of your life.

In a sense, therefore, it's best to start thinking about maintenance as soon as you begin your weight loss. If you can do that, you have substantially increased your chances of being in the small group of people who lose weight and keep it off. But the later you leave getting to grips with that thinking about new habits, the harder you are going to find the maintenance of your weight loss. And if you leave it until you have achieved your target weight and have started to maintain, keeping close to your target weight will be (just about) possible, but it will be a big and difficult job. And a job where few people succeed.

You may be thinking that *you* are now beginning maintenance and *you* have not acquired those beneficial habits, so what hope is there? As always, we can help, although there is no quick fix. If you did not start with parts 1 and 2 of the book, we suggest that it would be useful to read them now. This should not be too onerous because if you have reached your target weight without reading parts 1 and 2, then you clearly already have a lot of diet experience and have probably done many things right.

On the other hand, if you *did* start with parts 1 and 2, you may be feeling that you can proceed with confidence, but we still think that a refresher of at least slice 2 would be a good idea.

You may be interested in where *we* were in our weight-loss journey before we twigged that our dieting habits would have to carry on after reaching our target weights. The answer is that we were both just a few weeks before hitting our target weights. That may be why we have both had our fair share of maintenance difficulties, although we have generally handled those difficulties quite well. But then so we should – given all the thinking and work we have put into the book you are now holding!

**You hold onto your pre-diet idea of 'normal eating'**
How you were eating before you started to diet was either making you put on weight or making you maintain your weight at a higher level than you wanted to be. Either way, if you now go back to eating in that way, you will end up weighing – sooner or later – what you weighed before. You might remember this from slice 14:

If you eat what you always ate,<br>you'll weigh what you always weighed

So if you think of the way that you were eating before your diet started as 'normal eating', you are going to hit trouble in maintenance. And there is a particularly persuasive (hence dangerous) reason for you to think it is OK to go back to how you were eating before your diet started – you think that you deserve it.

It may seem perfectly reasonable, after working so hard to get down to your target weight, that you can reward yourself by going back to 'normal eating'. Unfortunately, the truth is that if you want to maintain your weight loss forever, 'normal eating' must become a way of eating that (1) you are happy to stick to and (2) keeps your weight where you want it to be.

For us, 'normal eating' still includes meals out, meals with friends, and holiday eating. But it is not the same as how we used to eat before our diets started – we now eat some different foods, and we usually eat a little less of everything. But this is not at all a hardship for us! We love what we eat nowadays. We have swapped our interests in baking cakes and eating frequent platefuls of cheese for new interests centred on discovering interesting, tasty, and low-calorie food.

**You get bored with the whole business of controlling your weight**
Many people find that they start off maintaining well, but then little things start to slip, their weight starts to increase, and they can't get it back under control. Keeping an eye on what they eat and what they weigh may not have the priority that it used to have, they become bored with the whole subject, and they get a feeling that maintaining is just not worth the effort. Then that old foe gets them – they get fed up and give up. More colourfully, they are experiencing weight control fatigue (an idea we introduced in slice 25).

It is simple weight control fatigue that is often behind why people – even after quite some time in maintenance – lose the battle and regain all of the weight they lost. Both of us have largely avoided weight control fatigue so far, so let's see some chat time on the subject:

*CHAT TIME*

*STEVE: Do you find it boring, always thinking about what you eat and keeping track of what you weigh?*

*CAROLINE: Not really, because I think back to when I was fat. I was always worrying about what I weighed and what I looked like and – in a sort of resigned way – what I was eating. Hardly a day would go by without thinking I should be limiting what I ate, and often in some minor way I would deprive myself of something.*

STEVE: *So you were always thinking about what you were eating, even when you were putting on weight or staying stable but obese?*

CAROLINE: *Yes, and feeling pretty rotten about it. There was often a voice in my head saying, 'You're so fat, you need to go on a diet, you're pathetic.'*

STEVE: *That doesn't sound much fun. What's different now you're maintaining at a healthy weight?*

CAROLINE: *Well, I still think about what I am eating, but much more positively. Nowadays, I think about what I weigh, but with pleasure and not shame. I still make choices about what I eat, but I am proud of the wise choices I make to stay a healthy weight. So I've swapped feeling bad about it all to feeling good about it all, and I've maintained my weight loss for longer than ever before.*

STEVE: *So it turns out that in maintenance you didn't have a choice between (1) thinking about what you ate and weighed and (2) giving in to weight control fatigue, giving up, and saving all that time by not thinking about it? There was no choice; you were going to think about it whatever you did.*

CAROLINE: *You're right. To put it more bluntly, I think my choice was 'Be fat and be unhappy about it – and think about it a lot' or 'Do something positive about maintaining a healthy weight, be slim, and be pleased about it – and think about it a lot.' Put like that, I much preferred (and still prefer) the second choice! What about you? Do you ever get weight control fatigue?*

STEVE: *No, not really. This whole question is simpler for me, because I have become so fascinated by the whole process of what I eat and how that affects my weight and health, I now call it a hobby and enjoy the time I spend thinking about it. Rather geekish, I know, so I don't really put myself forward as an example to follow – you are the shining example!*

*CAROLINE: You're too modest! I think it was you who applied the expression 'constant vigilance' to weight maintenance, the idea being that it is important for people who are maintaining to constantly have their diet and their weight in mind.*

*STEVE: True. Not necessarily to have them in mind with the same focus as while losing weight, but not forgetting about them either.*

*CAROLINE: And one of the reasons we both like the idea of constant vigilance is that there is strong evidence that most successful maintainers use constant vigilance. And we certainly do by, for example, keeping a close eye on what we eat and drink and by weighing ourselves often.*

Weight control fatigue is something that is most common when people have followed more restrictive diets, often because they hoped to lose weight quickly. If you have worked through the first half of this book, you will have noticed (especially in slice 16) that we believe that a good way to diet for the long term is to have a wide-ranging diet adapted to the realities of life. One of the reasons we think it's a good way to diet is because it's a way of making weight control fatigue less likely, hence making successful maintenance more likely.

However, if it's too late for that and you already feel bored and afflicted by weight control fatigue, do not despair! As we said above, the reason we wrote this book is to help you to learn to be in that small but happy band who lose weight and keep it off forever. So in slice 38 we will look at how to shake off weight control fatigue.

**You try to manage without the dieting techniques you learned while losing weight**
The fourth main reason why maintenance of weight loss can be difficult is that you get used to being at or around your target weight and start to take it for granted. You get complacent and feel that what you learned to do when you were slimming down to your target weight is all a bit of a nuisance and unnecessary for someone who is clearly at a good, healthy weight. You may even be encouraged to think like that by your friends and relatives, who might say things such as 'Why are you still on a diet? You've been slim for five years.'

You might be lucky and find that you can forget everything you learned about weight control and still maintain your target weight. But we think that is most unlikely. If it could happen like that, how did you manage to get overweight in the first place? So we think you should not abandon your good weight-loss habits. Particularly important are two points:

**It's risky to stop weighing yourself.** In slice 24 we wrote about the importance of weighing yourself while trying to lose weight. People often stop weighing themselves in maintenance. When they finally realise that all is not going well (maybe prompted by their tightening clothes) and they *do* weigh themselves, they can find they have put on a lot of weight. At the risk of repeating ourselves, they may then get fed up and give up. In slice 50, we will talk in more detail about stopping weighing yourself.

**It's risky to stop noticing what you eat.** What we mean by this is that while achieving a successful loss of weight, you were likely to have been taking an unusual interest in what you were eating and drinking. You may have been (1) counting calories, (2) thinking about whether you should be eating one food instead of another one, and (3) wondering whether you could 'afford' to eat something else late in the evening. And so on. Basically, you were taking a lot of notice of what you were eating and drinking. Once you have reached your target weight, your interest in the details of your food may have lessened. If that's true, you may be OK for a time, but gradually your weight may creep on as you increasingly slip back to what you used to eat without really noticing. So it is a good idea to keep at least some interest in the calories you are consuming.

Finally in this slice, if you find that your drive to maintain your target weight has simply evaporated and you are unsure what to do about it – we can offer you a quick fix! You could re-read part 2 of the book (slices 12–26, dealing with the specific actions to take in order to lose weight) and refresh your memory of them. That might highlight how much you have come to neglect those weight-loss actions and may inspire you to do some revision. That will make your start to maintenance so much easier.

# Slice 28

# Decide on your approach
to weight maintenance

Ideally, your approach to weight maintenance will take advantage of what you learned while losing weight and will help you through the transition from weight loss to weight maintenance and then forwards forever. This short slice offers some guidance on how these can be achieved.

Assuming that you are reading this having lost some weight, then it seems reasonable to think that you are generally happy with the way that you approached your weight loss (which we talked about in slice 6). We think that 'if it ain't broke, don't fix it' applies here – it may well be a good idea to stick to the general approach you adopted while losing weight. Of course, there will have to be some slight relaxation here and there so you don't continue to lose weight!

We think that taking similar approaches to both weight loss and weight maintenance helps you to realise that weight loss and maintenance are similar activities. One blends into the other. Although maintenance may be less intense, you still need to keep an eye on what you eat and what you weigh. We believe that maintenance needs such constant vigilance because without it, things may slip out of control (sometimes frighteningly quickly). Constant vigilance is an idea discussed further in slice 30.

If you do stick to a similar approach to both weight loss and weight maintenance, then there are several specific benefits. Those benefits accrue both during your period of transition from weight loss to maintenance and forwards into the many years of maintenance itself. The benefits include:

• You are more likely to hold onto your idea of 'normal eating', which you acquired while losing weight.
• You are more likely to continue with the eating habits you learned while losing weight.
• You are more likely to continue noticing what you eat.
• You are more likely to continue weighing yourself.

Despite these benefits, there is a potential problem that can arise in taking a similar approach to weight loss and weight maintenance. The issue is that because you are taking a similar approach, you will probably find that what you understood and what you did during weight loss is often closely related to what you have to understand and have to do during maintenance. You will notice this as you continue with the book – several slices suggest that you remember what you did during weight loss and 'keep at it'. That is generally a good thing, but the difficulty with keeping at it is that it can involve doing the same things for years. And doing the same things for years can lead to weight control fatigue – in other words, a lack of interest, causing various beneficial eating activities to slip over time. For now, this is simply to alert you to this possible downside of the 'keep at it' approach. You will come across 'weight control fatigue' many more times in the rest of the book, together with what to do about it.

There are further elements of how to approach your weight loss, which we discussed in slice 6. Briefly, those further elements concerned the complexity of your diet, your focus on exercise, how much planning to do, enlisting the help of others, and measuring your progress. You could consider which elements you will stick with in your life as a maintainer.

Finally in this slice, we think that there are two circumstances where carrying on into maintenance with your weight-loss approach may *not* be such a good idea. These circumstances are if you lost your weight quickly (1) on a very low-calorie diet (VLCD) or (2) on a latest-thing, attention-grabbing, celebrity-endorsed diet (often called a 'fad' diet).

    The problem with both types of diet is that they are difficult to stick to. You might have been able to follow one for a few weeks, but it is unlikely that you will still be following such a diet in a year, let alone in ten years. We suggest that if you did follow either type of fast-loss diet to achieve your target weight, you might consider another type of eating regime for maintenance. You may get some ideas about this in slice 6, in the section called 'What sort of diet will you follow?'

(Perhaps this is a good time to point out that the word 'diet' is often not quite correct when talking about maintenance. In everyday English, the word 'diet' is often used to mean a programme of weight reduction, which is usually more appropriate to weight loss. In the above paragraph, you will notice that we have used 'eating regime for maintenance' instead of 'diet' – that is more accurate, although less common. Such phrases will occur more and more in the remainder of the book.)

# Slice 29

# Those important first few weeks of maintenance

Slice 27 was a general introduction to your life as a 'maintainer', meaning someone who has lost weight and now wants to keep that weight off forever. We wanted to explain why maintenance was difficult, so it alerted you to the fact that maintenance needs to be taken seriously. We are now going to explain that not only are the points in slice 27 important, but they are pretty urgent too! That's because the single most dangerous time in your journey from being overweight to a lifetime of maintaining a good weight is immediately after you have reached your target weight.

This slice, therefore, highlights the importance of the very earliest days of maintenance. If you get that diet-into-maintenance transition wrong, it can cause unexpected problems with your maintenance. In the worst case, your maintenance can stall almost as soon as it has started – a huge pity after all of that work you put into losing weight. You'll be relieved to know that we have both experienced and worked through these transition problems ourselves and, yet again, we can help!

## Transition problem 1: there's little help on what to do when you hit target weight

Steve arrived at his target weight about a year before Caroline arrived at hers. He was amazed to find that there was almost no help available on what to do next – he found no books, few articles, and almost no search results on Google. A year later, Caroline found the same, with the exception of a blog by Steve. In fact, discussing that blog was one of our main inspirations to write the book you are now reading. To put it simply, you are virtually on your own unless (see slice 11) you have managed to find yourself a diet coach.

Our best guess at why there is this lack of help for the new maintainer is that nobody thinks that you have a problem. People may wonder *why* you should need help if you have managed to get down to your target weight. Hopefully slice 27 made that clear – because it is very difficult to maintain your target weight.

The snag is that because people have nowhere obvious to turn to for help, they do the most obvious thing they can think of and return to their pre-diet lifestyle. They may even be persuaded to do that by concerned friends and relatives who think they are already 'too thin'. The result of this was described in slice 27 – remember 'If you eat what you always ate, you'll weigh what you always weighed'? Fortunately, instead of that difficult situation, you have a book in your hands that will help you.

**Transition problem 2: those big celebrations on reaching your target weight**
For many people, losing weight (maybe a life-changing amount of weight) is a major achievement, and major achievements are often closely followed by major celebrations, involving eating and drinking. Neither of us is a stranger to such celebrations, and neither is Marianne, who is now maintaining after her large weight loss. So let's see some chat time that involved the three of us, illustrating the possible impact of celebrations on our weight.

*CHAT TIME*

STEVE: *Hello, Marianne. I know that you are successfully maintaining, but has that gone smoothly?*

MARIANNE: *It's going quite smoothly now, but I did have a real problem when I got to my target weight.*

CAROLINE: *Don't tell me – food and drink was involved.*

MARIANNE: *Oh yes! And the problem began on the exact day that I stepped on the scales and they showed my target weight of nine stone. It was a Friday morning, and by that evening my partner had organised a weekend break away.*

STEVE: *That's nice!*

MARIANNE: *Yes, it was. And although, deep down, I realised it was stupid, I ate and drank as much as I possibly could that weekend. After so much hard work and self-control, I felt as if I deserved it.*

*CAROLINE: I think we know where this is going – what did the scales say on Monday morning?*

*MARIANNE: They said that I had gained half a stone. I was really upset – I only lose weight slowly, and to get rid of that half a stone had probably taken me three whole months.*

*STEVE: But did you manage to lose that half stone, even if it did take a long time?*

*MARIANNE: No. I have a lot of lovely friends and family, and by the time we got back from the weekend away, they all seemed to know about me hitting my weight target. And by the time I went to bed, I was delighted to have a long list of parties and celebrations coming up in the following couple of weeks.*

*CAROLINE: That's fantastic!*

*MARIANNE: Err ... yes. But it meant that I didn't finish the final target-weight celebrations for ages. And when it all died down, I was well over a stone higher than my target weight.*

*CAROLINE: Oh dear. But looking at you now, I can see that you lost the weight you had put on.*

*MARIANNE: That's true, but it was not a good time for me. To cut a long story short, although I was majorly fed up and even thought about packing it all in, I did manage to get back to target weight eventually – but it took an eternity.*

We have heard stories like this many times. And, unlike Marianne, who had the dogged perseverance to get herself back to target weight in the end, many people don't manage it. They get fed up and give up, and not long afterwards, they are back to their original starting weight.

Someone (who didn't want her name to be mentioned in a book) sent us an email that is typical: 'Why do I do it every time?! I get to my target and feel like I've really achieved something. Then for no reason I eat and drink everything in sight. So mad with myself!! Does this happen to anyone else?? It's like my body or brain thinks *OK, you are where you want to be, so eat everything now – you've done what you wanted to do.*'

There are no figures we have seen concerning this, but it wouldn't surprise us if target-weight celebration was the number one cause of early weight maintenance failure.

There was more to the chat time as well.

## CHAT TIME

CAROLINE: So, Steve, what happened to you when you got to target weight?

STEVE: Ah yes, a very good question! I had followed a moderate weight-loss diet, and I well understood how getting to target weight would give me just 500 calories a day more than I had been consuming during weight loss. I knew I had to be careful!

MARIANNE: So how did it work out, clever clogs?

STEVE: Everything was fine just after reaching my target weight. But about six weeks after that, we went on a ten-day holiday. We were in a small town, but the town had three nice restaurants. I just ate what I wanted and returned home nine pounds heavier.

CAROLINE: Wow, nine pounds! I hope you immediately went back to careful eating.

STEVE. Sort of. I must say that I was worried for a time, but I did manage to re-establish some control, although it took a few weeks to lose that extra weight. But it did show me how easy it was to start regaining weight – even being confident of being right on top of things, and even some weeks after reaching target weight.

MARIANNE: What's your story, Caroline?

CAROLINE: My weight has drifted around a little since I started maintaining, but I have to say that I did not have any obvious upward leap just after getting to my target weight.

STEVE: Interesting. Caroline and I both had a similar good understanding of what we needed to do in that crucial time *after hitting our targets, and we had similar levels of motivation and willpower. But I had a problem and Caroline didn't.*

*CAROLINE: There's a good lesson to learn from all of our experiences. Maybe the best way of putting it is that the very start of maintenance is a dangerous time for everyone, that we all need to be alert, and that, whatever happens, we mustn't get fed up and give up.*

*MARIANNE: And haven't I also heard you two say that it is a bad idea to use food as reward?*

*CAROLINE and STEVE: Oh yes, that too! Thanks!*

**Transition problem 3: immediately going back to 'normal eating'**
We talked about this in slice 27, but it is worth repeating that you are now at a dangerous time in your journey to stay at a good weight forever. It is now that you need to fix in your mind that you cannot go back to eating as you did when you were overweight. And the reason we are saying this here, just after the chat time about target-weight celebrations, is that this is the most dangerous time of all. You need to form your good maintenance habits as early as possible, and the last thing you want instead is to put on a lot of celebration weight.

But let's assume that any celebrations finished without a big gain, and let's also assume that you are clear about not going back to how you were eating before your diet started. That's a great start to maintenance, but what now? Many people are unsure what to do next, especially because (as we saw earlier) there is not much help on the subject.

Our advice is not to throw away all that you have learned about weight loss by starting some completely different maintenance eating regime. Instead, decide to build on your successful weight-loss eating and simply carry on with that into maintenance, with some tweaks. And do that immediately you reach your target weight.

The tweaked version we suggest is to begin your maintenance by adding (let's say) 300 calories a day to what you allowed yourself while losing weight. After a month, have a look at how your weight compares to what it was when you started to maintain. There are three possible results:

• Your weight is unchanged. So stick with the 300 calories a day.

• Your weight is still going down. You need to eat some more calories, so increase your 'maintenance bonus' to (say) 400 calories a day.

• Your weight is going up. You need to eat slightly fewer calories, so reduce your bonus to (say) 200 calories a day.

A month later, have another look at how your weight is moving (if at all). Adjust your bonus again if necessary. You get the idea. But take it easy – don't change your maintenance bonus every day! You have plenty of time to get the bonus just right, so you are neither losing nor gaining. And don't worry too much – many people are concerned that they will increase their calories a little and suddenly put on those pounds that they worked hard to lose. But if you are adjusting by only slightly too much, it will take you weeks to gain even a pound.

# Slice 30

# Get motivated and stay motivated
# in maintenance

In slice 3, we said that motivation is at the heart of any attempt to lose weight and keep that weight off. Without motivation, your weight loss and your maintenance may well be doomed to failure. Motivation is clearly extremely important!

We covered various aspects of motivation in slice 3 – what motivation is, why it matters, how to get motivated, how to stay motivated, and how to keep your motivation thriving when things go wrong. All of these are still important in maintenance, although there are now some further points to make about how to stop your motivation from weakening.

During weight loss, many of us find that our motivation decreases as time goes on. But our own experience, and what we have heard from many other maintainers, suggests that a drop-off of motivation is probably even more of a problem during maintenance. This is hardly surprising given that motivation to lose weight usually needs to last for a reasonably short time but motivation to *maintain* weight often needs to last for decades. And the excitement of weight loss cannot be matched by the quiet satisfaction of staying the same, year after year!

We think that the main possible reasons that motivation reduces in maintenance are:

• Believing that the difficulties of losing weight will carry on forever.
• Just not wanting to be bothered with dieting forever.
• Believing that the compliments received about weight loss will dry up.

We have some good news! Although there is a little truth in these beliefs, they are nothing like as bad as you might think, and there are motivation-boosting positives that can be taken from all of them. So let's investigate them one at a time.

**Believing that the difficulties of losing weight will carry on forever**
As we have said before, losing weight is difficult. So as people approach maintenance, they can be demotivated if they think that such difficulty is going to continue far into the future. But we are pleased to give you the good news that, in some ways, *maintenance does get easier*. It gets

easier because you get more and more used to doing what you need to do. Let's have a look at our own experiences.

## CHAT TIME

*STEVE: I think we both feel that life gets a little easier after some time in maintenance.*

*CAROLINE: Yes, that's true. I think it's largely a matter of keeping at it – like many things in life, the more you do something, the easier it gets. So, for example, if you keep going with small permanent changes [covered in slice 13], then they just become habits, and no trouble at all.*

*STEVE: That's definitely the case for me – I have always been a fan of SPCs, and those that I have been doing for years are now just part of my life.*

*CAROLINE: Like what?*

*STEVE: I think that a big calorie-saver for me has been to have skimmed milk rather than semi-skimmed or even full-fat milk. At first skimmed milk tasted strange, but after a couple of weeks I didn't really notice it, and after some months I had some semi-skimmed milk in a cup of tea and I didn't like it at all. Now, after some years, having skimmed milk is effortless – it's just totally normal. And I benefit from hundreds of other such effortless SPCs.*

*CAROLINE: That's a good example. So although setting up SPCs during weight loss does take some effort, if you succeed, maintenance will become easier – you will rely less on motivation and more on habit (always a powerful driver of behaviour).*

*STEVE: Even better, the more you become used to eating in this new way, the more you come to like it and the easier it becomes. This may sound magical, but it's been true for both of us. And there are many other ways that maintenance can get easier, which have nothing to do with SPCs.*

*CAROLINE: Yes, a good example is BOGOFs. It is easy to be*

*impressed by them [see slice 15]. But once, during weight loss, you see why you need to be wary of a BOGOF, you'll always understand why. So it will be easier to be careful about BOGOFs in maintenance.*

Those examples illustrate how, once you get used to something in maintenance, it often needs little or no effort to keep it going. And that is *motivating* – not the opposite! In fact, this process of putting work into making required changes, then having them under your belt forever applies to pretty much everything we covered in the first two parts of the book.

Another thought that you may find as motivating as we do is that if you have got through the difficulties of weight loss and succeeded in reaching your target weight, you are a person in control of your weight. We certainly found it a great feeling – after all of those years of yo-yo dieting and of generally feeling powerless to stop the yo-yoing, we were finally in control. A powerful motivator!

**Just not wanting to be bothered with dieting forever**
We have been talking about how maintenance is not all that difficult – assuming that good practice was learned during weight loss. We find that to be motivating, and we know others do too. But for some people the problem is not so much the difficulty or otherwise of maintenance, it is what they see as the whole tedious business of 'being on a diet forever'. They find it demotivating to have to pay attention to their eating regime and their weight for many years to come.

It is important to talk this through because if you are demotivated by being careful about your eating in maintenance, then you may switch back to eating what you ate before your weight-loss diet started. And 'if you eat what you always ate, you'll weigh what you always weighed' may apply.

Research suggests that some (lucky) people are unable to become overweight. But, in our modern society, people who are *able* to become overweight usually *do* become overweight. So if you have been overweight, then you slimmed down to target weight, you are probably stuck with the tendency to become overweight again. And you are going to have to work against that tendency for the rest of your life by controlling your weight.

Your only choices in maintenance (other than the unappealing one of staying overweight forever) are therefore:

**Start to yo-yo diet.** In other words, (1) gain weight (maybe a lot), (2) lose weight to get back to your target weight, and (3) repeat. At any one time, you will either be gaining weight (and probably not liking it) or trying to lose weight (and probably feeling pretty fed up with yourself and with the whole business of dieting). If you follow this path, then you will often be thinking about what you eat and what you weigh.

OR

**Keep your weight roughly at your target weight.** Having a stable weight has benefits. You will probably be healthier and fitter, and you won't have to keep clothes of different sizes. You also may be feeling a little bit pleased with yourself! If you follow this path, then you will often be thinking about what you eat and what you weigh.

You will immediately notice that, *whichever you choose*, you will have to spend a lot of time thinking about what you eat and what you weigh! So if you want to control your weight forever, then, unfortunately, not bothering with your eating regime is not an option.

The option you *do* have is whether to yo-yo diet or stay at roughly the same weight. It's a personal choice, but our view is that yo-yo dieting is hard work and carries the risk of getting fed up. We have seen many people whose weight has yo-yoed, but they all eventually returned to their pre-weight-loss weight (or higher). So our choice of how to control *our* weight for life is certainly to try to stick close to our target weight forever.

Being careful forever may not have been what you had in mind when you set off to lose weight – weeks, months, or years ago. What you might have thought of as a 'diet for life' may not have been an attractive idea then and may not be now. But if it's not an attractive idea, we can offer you some motivation to be careful forever. That motivation is that it is well-established that most successful long-term maintainers *do* keep a keen interest in their calories, *do* weigh themselves often, and *do* keep their weight fairly stable. So you will be increasing your chances of being in that elite.

And you may be even more motivated because there are some in that elite who seem to get a feel for what they should and shouldn't consume, and they don't need to think about it very much. They are the lucky 'naturally slim' people – the happy band that Steve referred to back in slice 13. Joining that band would be the pinnacle of dieting!

**Believing that the compliments received about weight loss will dry up**

Not everyone seems to be interested in what people say about their new and slimmer form. But many are, and they will have found the positive comments highly motivating while they were losing weight. So, to those who do find nice comments motivating: we really understand what a big task that weight loss was and encourage you to feel very pleased with yourself. Because – and here is the sad part – on the whole, the positive comments from others will peter out soon, if they haven't already. So we're afraid that you will need to accept that that feeling of being pleased will be generated by yourself! There may be exceptions, as we talked about in another chat.

### CHAT TIME

*STEVE: I only got to know you after you had arrived at your target weight – did your body change dramatically enough to get a lot of comments while you were losing weight?*

*CAROLINE: Yes, I did lose a considerable percentage of my body weight, and the change was easily noticeable. But once I started to maintain, there was just the occasional comment, mostly about how long I had managed to keep my weight off. Although I am still amused and delighted by the comment that was made to me after about six months of maintenance by a new (overweight) colleague: 'Have you always been slim?'*

*STEVE: But would you say that the compliments you received in maintenance motivated you?*

*CAROLINE: Yes, I would – it may have been only a trickle, but it was a motivating trickle! And I will probably remember that 'always been slim' comment for years. It did make me think that whenever I meet one of those rare people who has lost weight and kept it off, I should make sure that I am as complimentary as I possibly can be. So what sort of comments did you get?*

*STEVE: I suppose that my weight loss was even more dramatic. I nearly halved my body weight and went from being very fat indeed to quite slim. Because of that, I got a lot of positive feedback while losing weight.*

*CAROLINE: Did that then reduce to a trickle when maintaining, as mine did?*

*STEVE: Actually, for a long time, no. Because of the nature of my work, I sometimes don't see people for some years, so I had a continuous stream of people who hadn't seen me since I lost weight. They were suitably impressed, and I was suitably motivated! And, best of all, I have had four (yes, I am counting them!) excellent experiences of people not even recognising me because I had lost so much weight.*

*CAROLINE: And don't forget that we have also been asked on several occasions how we managed to lose weight and how we managed to keep it off. That is also motivating, as well as being one of the reasons to write our book on the subject!*

So our experiences of feedback in maintenance are something of a mixed bag – they depend to some extent on what we do in our different lives. But we have both had really good and motivational experiences, even years after reaching target weight. Wonderful as they are, however, these experiences are probably not frequent enough to be relied on: we (and you) must also keep up motivation from within. So we are now going to look at a further idea to maintain motivation in maintenance.

## Constant vigilance

We said earlier in this slice that, for most people who are maintaining after being overweight, you will need to be careful forever. We often call this exercising 'constant vigilance'. People can find constant vigilance depressing and demotivating, but we both find constant vigilance actively *motivating*. Let's look at some chat time between ourselves and Natasha about this interesting mental about-turn.

*CHAT TIME*

*CAROLINE: I know that you recently lost over five stone – well done!*

*NATASHA: Thanks! But I do worry about maintenance – I have heard you and Steve talking about having to keep an eye on things for a long, long time. I'd much prefer just to get on with my life.*

STEVE: Yes, I did find the idea of constant vigilance a little hard to come to terms with, but Caroline showed me another way of thinking about it. Caroline – the floor is yours!

CAROLINE: I did think that it might not be much fun to be constantly vigilant. But then I asked myself what would happen if I lost my grip and went back to being overweight? I remembered that being overweight is not much fun either. And it is not exciting to feel frumpy and wear clothes because they hide the bulges and because you can fit into them – rather than because you like the look of them.

NATASHA: Yes, I remember that well.

CAROLINE: And there's more. How interesting is it to be told (directly or through hints) that you need to lose weight? How fascinating is it to brood about your weight? How refreshing is it to be out of breath walking even a short distance? And how uplifting is it to catch a glimpse of yourself in a shop window and think how fat you are?

STEVE: Yes indeed. In summary, is it a good experience to be overweight? I certainly didn't find it so.

NATASHA: And neither did I. Not for a minute.

CAROLINE: So then I made the mental step of thinking that, compared to the downsides of being overweight, keeping a constant eye on my weight and what I eat is not at all depressing. In fact, it is liberating! I am no longer at the mercy of my weight – I am in control of it. I know that constant vigilance is all I need to do to ensure that I never go back to being fat again! What's not to like?

NATASHA: Wow, you certainly know something about motivation. I think what I should do is to write a list of what I hated about being five stone heavier. In other words, everything that I really, really don't want to go back to!

STEVE: And I would add to it what you can do now that you never imagined you would be able to do again.

*NATASHA: Yes, you're right. I've started to play badminton again, and I haven't been able to do that for over twenty years.*

*CAROLINE: And write these things down now, before you get so used to them that you stop appreciating them! Then – one last thought – dig out your list from time to time, read it carefully, and think that all you need to do in order to keep those wonderful changes you have made is stay vigilant. That's pure motivation!*

We have two last thoughts before finishing this slice.

• That last chat time was basically about shifting your thinking. Another useful shift – even while dieting – is to think of the long-term benefits of keeping that weight off. If, early in our weight-loss journey, we can devote some of our thinking to the long term, then we lessen the chances of allowing ourselves to eat in an unhelpful manner when we reach target weight.

• If you are the type of person who finds numbers motivating (certainly we both are), then you probably liked to see the number on the scales going down while losing weight. That motivation is no longer there in maintenance, or at least the buzz of staying the same week after week after week is a particularly modest little buzz! An alternative way of being motivated by numbers in maintenance would be good, and you may be able to think of how to do that. But if not, Steve came up with a system that motivates him well, and it may help you to. We will cover this later in the book (in slice 50).

# Slice 31

# Understand emotional eating
# in maintenance

Slice 4 was about gaining an understanding of emotional eating while losing weight, and we hope that was useful in getting down to your target weight. As you now move into the maintenance of your weight loss, there are some further issues that you will benefit from understanding. Let's begin by considering three groups.

- **Non-emotional eaters.** People who slimmed down to their target weight without ever experiencing emotional eating. They are the lucky ones, and we are going to assume that they will carry on eating, unaffected by their emotions.
- **Ex-emotional eaters.** People who were emotional eaters, who read and understood what we wrote earlier about understanding emotional eating (slice 4), then followed our advice about handling that emotional eating (slice 20) – and slimmed down to their target weight. This slice is written for these ex-emotional eaters because over the many years of maintenance, they may find that their emotional eating returns.
- **Still-emotional eaters.** People who were emotional eaters, read and understood everything we wrote, but didn't follow our advice (no hard feelings, though!). They carried on being emotional eaters and nevertheless still managed to reach their target weight. We would guess that there are not many people in this category because, in our experience, people who are emotional eaters find it particularly difficult to lose weight. This slice is also written for those still-emotional eaters, because they may find that the impact of their emotional eating grows and leads to weight gain.

To ex-emotional eaters and still-emotional eaters, we are going to repeat the stark and (sorry!) unamusing message we gave to you in slice 4. That message was that you have a choice to make. The emotions and experiences driving you to eat unhelpfully may be very strong, very sad, very deep. Your choice, however, is either (1) to use the emotions as an excuse not to lose weight or (2) to find a way to tackle them because you want to stay at a healthy weight. The toughest bit is that if you are eating emotionally, sooner or later it is likely to get in the way of long-term maintenance of your weight loss.

There are areas of dieting where it is possible to ease off once you arrive at maintenance – for example, once you get to your target weight, you can increase (at least a little) the number of calories you consume. Unfortunately, emotional eating is not one of those areas – with emotional eating there can be little or no easing off in maintenance. Easing off to become more of an emotional eater has the potential for causing rapid weight gain, which is discouraging (maybe even disastrous). Remember that anything that can trip you up in dieting can trip you up in maintenance. So we suggest that a good start to maintenance is to have another look at slices 4 and 20.

Having revised those slices and once more become an 'expert', then you 'only' have to 'keep at it'! However, although 'keep at it' works well for many aspects of maintenance, it may not succeed as well for emotional eating. Lives rarely stay exactly the same forever, and changes in the life of an emotional eater may quickly lead to emotional changes and to overeating. It is a good idea to be alert to such changes in eating habits so you can take action as soon as possible, and certainly before a weight gain becomes so big that even you – a successful dieter and maintainer – get fed up and give up.

For the rest of this slice, we are going to revisit three issues we discussed in slice 4 – issues where weight control fatigue can develop and become a problem in maintenance. But we do suggest that while you are looking at slice 4, it would be a good idea to think about this for yourself. By the time we meet up in slice 46 (about how to actually handle emotional eating in maintenance), we will be able to compare notes!

One issue we talked about in slice 4 was **how to be sure whether you emotionally overeat or not**. We suggested that it might help to ask yourself two questions about the last time you overate:
'Were you content, involved in what you were doing, or in pleasant company?' That sounds as if it *wasn't* emotional eating.
'Were you bored, lonely, sad, angry, frustrated, scared, or any combination of these?' That sounds as if it *was* emotional eating.

It is a good idea to occasionally ask yourself those two questions to test whether your emotional eating is on the rise.

Those questions may not be conclusive. But, as we said above, your life is unlikely to stay exactly the same forever, and emotional changes will probably happen at some time. If they are not changes for the better, you may feel that emotional eating is creeping back into your life. If you do, you may need to refer to slice 46 for ideas about how to handle it.

We also said in slice 4 that if you are a spur-of-the-moment emotional eater, it is useful to **know which emotions trigger your eating** so you can do something about it. Again, forever is a long time, and the lives of most people change, so it is (constant vigilance again) a good idea to keep an eye on the emotions that trigger your overeating. Those triggering emotions may be different from those you experienced in the past – possibly years ago.

The third point we made in slice 4 was that if you are a longstanding emotional eater and, while losing weight, **you managed the difficult task of consciously changing a deeply ingrained habit**, then that was an achievement to be proud of. But in maintenance, it is useful to be alive to the possibility that your achievement may begin to backslide. It may *seem* that you have changed deeply ingrained habits, but some habits can be *so* deeply ingrained that they have a nasty habit of resurfacing. If the deeply ingrained habits do resurface, it is important to recognise that fact and try to do something about it. And the quicker the better, because the longer the deeply ingrained habits are re-established, the harder they will be to shift.

This slice has been about understanding emotional eating in maintenance. Slice 46 builds on that understanding and discusses what you can actually do about it.

# Slice 32

# Beware of self-defeating thoughts in maintenance

In slice 5, we looked at the problem of self-defeating thoughts – thoughts that stop you from getting on with your dieting the way you want to. We saw that these self-defeating thoughts can seriously interfere with your weight-loss plans, and we talked you through a five-point approach to successfully addressing them. Now that you are maintaining your weight, the problem of self-defeating thoughts may still be around, and you will need to deal with them and keep dealing with them forever.

You saw in slice 5 how powerful self-defeating thoughts are. If you are frequently a victim of such thoughts, there is a risk that you may give up your diet. But if you are reading this now, it seems likely that you achieved your target weight, and so had some success at dealing with self-defeating thoughts. Well done!

There will be some self-defeating thoughts that you countered so often, and so successfully, that countering them became a habit and, in the end, you didn't even think about them. For example, if every single time you overdid the calories on Friday evening you immediately got back in control on Saturday morning. In that way, you countered the self-defeating thought 'I'll leave it until Monday', and immediately getting back in control just became 'what you did' – you no longer needed any great willpower to do it. That is good. That is very good. But (yes, we know, there's always a but!) ...

There may be other self-defeating thoughts that have proved more difficult for you, and you *still* wrestle with them in maintenance. Perhaps you still have a great liking for chocolate biscuits, and you get the self-defeating thought that you need to keep a supply handy in case the grandchildren pop in for a visit. (Unfortunately, you find that you need to keep restocking the cupboard – because you end up eating them yourself!) In more difficult cases like that, you need to keep working on dealing with the self-defeating thought, and we hope you will be able to use the five-point approach we described in slice 5.

This is an important matter because you are in it for the long haul now, and any self-defeating thoughts you do *not* deal with may, over time, lead to another self-defeating thought, and then another one. Eventually you will be back to making a lot of excuses as your weight gets higher and higher. But remember: these old self-defeating thoughts are thoughts you did tackle at one time, even if there has been some backsliding. You know something about the thoughts and may now be better able to deal with them successfully. These old self-defeating thoughts are nevertheless an issue, but there is a further issue too: you may start to hear some *new* self-defeating thoughts. We are going to look at two particularly difficult examples of self-defeating thoughts that can pop up for long-term maintainers.

- 'My weight is stable – maybe I no longer need to be so careful about what I eat.'
- 'I might have become one of those "naturally slim" people. I can eat what I like now.'

It would be a good idea to practise using that five-point approach to understand how to deal with both of the new self-defeating thoughts above. But, to help you, we are now going to look at some more detail about them, as we discussed in a chat time.

### CHAT TIME

*CAROLINE: Let's begin with the self-defeating thought 'My weight is stable – maybe I no longer need to be careful about what I eat.'*

*STEVE: It's easy to understand why this self-defeating thought might occur. People you have met recently may never have seen the 'overweight you'. In fact, a lot of people have said to me, 'I can't believe you were ever overweight.'*

*CAROLINE: Yes, that's the same for me. And also, if you have been maintaining for a long time, even people you have known since the days when you were overweight may have simply forgotten that 'old you'. You may have even forgotten the 'old you' yourself unless you look at some old photographs.*

*STEVE: I know that when I look at old photographs, it doesn't really feel as if I am looking at myself.*

*CAROLINE: And that all adds up to a problem – if nobody thinks of you as an overweight person (not even yourself!) – then it becomes hard to believe that you need to watch what you eat or do anything special at all. And the longer you maintain, the harder it gets to believe it.*

STEVE: And that's when a self-defeating thought such as 'My weight is stable – maybe I no longer need to be careful about what I eat' can start getting louder.

CAROLINE: I suppose the key to this particular self-defeating thought is not to believe it automatically.

STEVE: Yes, maybe you no longer need to be quite so careful. But you do need to keep checking how you are actually doing – by weighing yourself. If your weight is going up, that is the time to go back to doing everything you learned while losing weight. I think that is key to it – you can believe whatever you want as long as you have the occasional reality check.

CAROLINE: Let's have a look now at another self-defeating thought – 'I might have become one of those "naturally slim" people. I can eat what I like now.' This is an even more optimistic self-defeating thought than the first! If you believe that you are one of those 'naturally slim' people, then you can certainly persuade yourself that you can eat what you like. [The subject of 'naturally slim' people is also covered in slice 30.]

STEVE: I think this thought is a particularly risky one because if it were true, then there would indeed be no need to control eating and drinking at all.

CAROLINE: Sometimes, you do hear that so-and-so can eat and eat and never put on a pound. Even if it's true, it's probably because they are blessed with the 'right genes'. If someone used to be overweight then, even if they slimmed down, they cannot have those 'right genes', and they never will have – you can't acquire new genes.

STEVE: And recent thinking is that, with a very few exceptions, 'naturally slim' people are just people like all the rest of us, but they have learned to be careful about what they eat. If they eat a bit too much, then the next day they eat less to compensate. They always control what they consume – and that's what we need to do as well.

CAROLINE: In any case, even if someone is totally convinced

*that they are 'naturally slim', then, as you said earlier, they need to check that this is true by weighing themselves regularly.*

That chat also covered similar ground to the common maintainers' self-defeating thought: 'It's unfair – why do I have to diet for my whole life when others don't?' That one is so common that we used it as an example of our five-point approach in slice 5. As you can probably spot very quickly, the reason it's not unfair is because most people who keep to a good body weight are simply paying attention to what they eat. They just may not call it a 'diet', because that is just their usual way of eating.

Remember that, in maintenance, you are faced with trying to counter self-defeating thoughts forever. And these are not just self-defeating thoughts you already know about but new self-defeating thoughts that may appear, possibly many years after reaching target weight. You need to use constant vigilance (and our five-point approach) against them all!

# Slice 33

## Decide on your long-term goal and at what point you will have 'strayed' from that goal

We do understand that your journey from starting to diet to achieving your target weight may have been eventful and difficult. If you are now maintaining, however, you must have achieved something amazing – you must have decided on a target weight, and you must have kept going until you hit that target weight.

Maintenance is different. The idea of maintenance is that you will be keeping your weight under control forever. But forever is a long time, and over that long time, many things can happen in our lives. Maybe we will get an illness that needs us to change our diet a lot. Maybe we will take up marathon running or injure ourselves so we can no longer exercise much. And, anyway, as the years wear on, a normal slowing of our metabolism (see slice 51) tends to lead to slight weight increase. In brief, we believe that we need to be flexible about long-term goals.

Flexibility in long-term goals can take many forms. As examples:
• You simply might want to set a long-term goal that is higher (or lower) than the target weight you slimmed down to.
• Rather than setting a long-term goal that is a fixed weight, you might want to have an 'acceptable weight band'.
• You might want to set a long-term goal for the next (let's say) three years and once those three years are up, think about whether changing circumstances mean you want to change that goal for the following three years.

Let's look at how flexibility in long-term goals worked for us.

### CHAT TIME

*STEVE: Would you say that there was flexibility in your long-term goal?*

*CAROLINE: Yes, but not so much to begin with. When I got to my dieting target weight, I just assumed that I would try to stay roughly at that weight forever. But I did cut myself a little slack and set what I thought was an acceptable weight band from four pounds below my dieting target weight to three pounds above.*

*STEVE: And have you kept within that band ever since?*

*CAROLINE: Not exactly. Changes do happen in life, and you wouldn't expect to focus on body weight quite as much in maintenance as when trying to lose weight. So I have occasionally drifted above and below that band. But generally, my weight has been on an even keel. How about you?*

*STEVE: I also set an acceptable weight band, but my weight tends to bob up and down more than yours, so my band was wide – five pounds below to five pounds above my target weight. I also stayed flexible about what my long-term goal might be.*

*CAROLINE: Why did you want to do that?*

*STEVE: Because after beginning maintenance, I continued to lose weight slowly – about a stone in the first three years. Then I thought that weight was too low, so I gradually (and very carefully!) allowed it to drift up a little. So it took me several years to be sure of what I wanted my long-term weight goal to be.*

*CAROLINE: What we both did, and both thought was most important, was to continue weighing ourselves regularly.*

*STEVE: Yes indeed. If you don't know what is happening to your weight, it's hard to tell whether things are moving in the wrong direction, and hence whether you need to do something about it.*

From that chat, it's clear that we like the idea of some flexibility in long-term goals. But we are always careful not to misuse the idea of 'flexibility'. We don't like using flexibility as an excuse to ignore warning signs, as in the following examples:

- 'My weight is OK – my clothes aren't any tighter.'
- 'My weight is OK – I looked too scrawny before.'
- 'My weight is OK – I'm still three stone lighter than I used to be.'
- 'My weight is OK – this extra weight is OK; it's a better weight for winter.'

The snag with being flexible is that (especially if you are good at making excuses!) things can drift out of control, and the next time you look at the scales you have put on a lot of weight and get fed up. You know what can happen then – you give up. So we think that an important tool for a successful maintainer is to have a weight that is a red line. If you get as high as that red line, there are no ifs, buts, or maybes – you have strayed, and you must do something about it.

But what should your red line be? That's up to you, but we suggest

• it shouldn't be too low. If it is, you will always be pressing the 'panic button' even if you've only put on the odd pound, and

• it shouldn't be too high. If it is, you might have put on so much that it seems a huge task to bring it down again.

To give you an idea, we both have red lines, and they are more than half a stone higher than our long-term goals. At the time of writing, we have both got to our red lines once, realised we had strayed, then lost weight to come back to where they should be – the safety net worked!

There is something else we are going to cover concerning red lines. The problem discussed in the chat time below may not concern many people, but for those who are affected, it is of great importance.

### CHAT TIME

CAROLINE: *We talked about a red-line weight we would absolutely not go above. But what about a weight we would not go below? For a lot of people, that is the least of their worries – what they are keen to do is not put on too much weight. But it's true that some people have the opposite problem.*

STEVE: *Typically, they settle into a comfortable new lifestyle while they are losing weight and once they get to their target weight, they never really stop 'dieting'. So their weight continues to fall.*

CAROLINE: *And that can be dangerous.*

STEVE: *Yes. And I have had a taste of that problem. As I said earlier, my weight continued to drift down slowly in my first three years of maintenance, and both my wife and diet coach suggested that I needed to set myself a low-weight red line.*

CAROLINE: *They certainly did, but there was quite a lot of drama before that actually happened.*

STEVE: *Yes indeed. It was surprisingly difficult to stop my weight loss. My problem was that I had followed a pretty strict regime for the best part of two years and achieved something that was (for me) amazing. I was worried that once I stopped that regime so that I could gain a little weight, I might then find that the wind changed and I would be unable to stop gaining. I'm not a particularly anxious type, but I was genuinely frightened.*

CAROLINE: *I do understand that, and I have heard quite a few people say something similar. So what did you do about it?*

STEVE: *What I did first was recognise how risky the weight gain would be. I was going to deliberately put on weight for the first time in my life. And then I was going to try to stop exactly when I wanted to stop.*

CAROLINE: *You were right to identify how difficult it was going to be to stop gaining. You had had decades of practice at gaining weight, and the risk was that those old habits would quickly re-establish themselves. So how did you tackle the problem?*

STEVE: *I began by setting myself a target weight (this time to be approached from below). Then I decided not to change my new, successful weight-loss habits but just add in some 'extras'. But I was careful to make them extras that I would be able to stop having.*

CAROLINE: *How did you know which extras you would be able to turn off like that?*

STEVE: *That was the clever bit! I did not add in foods that I had learned from dieting experience that I had little control over. Cheese, for example. Or bread. Instead my extras were foods that I was not particularly fond of. People did think this was an odd approach, but it seemed like a good one to me. I added in foods such as nuts and some starters, such as garlic bread and olives.*

*CAROLINE: That's interesting. You based your approach on what you knew about your own eating likes and then problem-solved to find a solution. But a solution that many others might find useful.*

*STEVE: Yes, and the final idea was (in the same way as losing weight) not to gain weight too quickly. I think it took me a month to gain the six pounds to reach my target. And it was easy for me to stop those occasional extras – I never really liked them much anyway!*

*CAROLINE: Everything turned out well, and your diet coach did then persuade you that it was a good idea to set a low-weight red line.*

*STEVE: It was easy to persuade me, and it has been useful because since then, I have again seen the low-weight red line approaching. I have upped my calories in the same way as before until I got back to my long-term goal.*

Finally, while reading this slice, you may have been wondering what you can do if your goals are not in terms of body weight. We discussed this earlier in the book (in slice 6), where we said that our book is primarily focused on measuring body weight. We recognise that some people prefer targets that are not in stones and pounds – they prefer targets such as waist measurement, dress size, or simply looking good. We said that the advantage of measuring in stones and pounds is that it is reasonably precise, and usually more precise than waist size, dress size, or how good you look. But, on the other hand, anything that people find helpful has to be all to the good, so you can re-read this slice, substituting the measurement of your choice for 'weight'. Whatever the measurement of your choice is, however, we suggest you measure it fairly often, and make it as accurate as you can.

# Slice 34

# Understand the benefits of counting and recording calories in maintenance

If you are reading this, you may well have achieved your target weight, quite possibly by using the system that we believe gives the best chance of success. That system – the one that we followed and that we discussed in slice 8 – is to give yourself an allowance of calories you can consume every day, then to keep a running total of how many calories you have left for that day.

Our experience, and that of a lot of other successful dieters, is that operating such a system in order to get to target weight is fairly hard work for a week or two, but then it quickly becomes easier, just like any other routine. So, in general, doing it is not a problem. And – in principle – it continues not to be a problem during maintenance. But, in reality, how you feel about following 'the system' can change during those long years of maintenance, and we discussed this in some chat time.

*CHAT TIME*

*CAROLINE: Let's start by touching on how our system of keeping track of calories consumed against a daily allowance worked during weight loss. Then we can talk about what changed once we moved into maintenance.*

*STEVE: OK. After getting into the swing of that system right at the start of your diet, how much of your day did you spend operating the system?*

*CAROLINE: On most days, it was no more than five minutes. The occasional resetting of my allowance took next to no time; weighing of what I was eating and drinking was quick (and for many food items, the weight was already on the packet).*

*STEVE: Did you also need to check the calories in foods you had never eaten before?*

*CAROLINE: Oh yes. I didn't want to make the rookie error of getting used to enjoying something new and then finding out that it was high in calories. But checking those calories was just an occasional job. And, finally, recording in an online food diary was no hardship.*

*STEVE: That seems a real success story. Are you still doing calorie counting now that you are some years into maintenance?*

*CAROLINE: Yes, I am. In maintenance, I have carried on recording what I consume and the calories they contain in just the same way as when I was losing weight.*

*STEVE: But I do have the impression that your maintenance system is still slightly more relaxed than the system under which you lost your weight.*

*CAROLINE: You're right. If the system under which I lost my weight could be called the 'full' system, you could call mine the 'slightly light' system. For example, I find that I can now afford to estimate calories a little more often than when I was losing weight, and I can have the occasional unrecorded biscuit – that sort of thing. I like to think that the many good habits I acquired during weight loss mean that a few relaxations in the 'full' system are acceptable in maintenance.*

*STEVE: That seems like a good continuation of your success story. I think my journey has also been successful, but I haven't followed the 'full' system quite as closely as you did.*

*CAROLINE: So what did you do that was different?*

*STEVE: Well, at the start of my diet, I did everything just so. But after about a year I found a way of eating where it was fairly easy for me to stay within my calorie allowance on most days, and I also got good at estimating the weight of what I was eating. So I thought I might be able to stop my calorie counting without ill effects by using my own relaxed system.*

*CAROLINE: But why stop? Why not carry on with a system that was working well?*

*STEVE: It's a long time ago now, but I seem to remember reading a message board post where someone was saying what a nuisance it was to keep completing a food diary. I wondered how I would find it when I finally got to maintaining, and I thought I would experiment to see whether I could stop completing my food diary – but still control my weight.*

*CAROLINE: Weren't you worried that all of your good work would unravel?*

*STEVE: Yes, very worried! But I did keep on weighing myself, and every day too. And my version of the system worked for me – it worked during weight loss and it continues to work during maintenance. I think that if your version of the system was called the 'slightly light' system, you could probably think of mine as the 'very light' system.*

*CAROLINE: It's not so surprising that we had different approaches. It's because my situation was different from yours – I am a small and light woman, and so I have a lower calorie allowance. My everyday careful eating is quite close to the daily calories at which I would put weight on, so I have to be more vigilant than you. Did you ever actually go back to calorie counting?*

*STEVE: Yes. I sometimes go back to weighing and recording everything – the 'full' system. It is especially useful after events like holidays where, if I have put on a little weight and I want to be absolutely sure of getting rid of that weight, I can get back on track. I think that reduces my stress because I keep my hand in with the 'full' system, and I know that I can always return to it.*

We think that this chat neatly illustrates the points we particularly want to get across to you in this slice:
• Counting calories forever is, for some people, not difficult. For such people, it can be a good path to follow.
• If you don't want to count calories forever, then a 'lighter' version of the system of counting and recording calories against a target allowance might be good enough for maintenance. You may find that habits you acquired during weight loss will be successful enough for you to be able

to maintain under a 'lighter' system. We're thinking of habits such as mainly cooking from scratch, keeping to a low-fat (or low-sugar) diet, only eating bread and potatoes at the weekend, etc., etc., etc.

• Even if you are going to be more informal about controlling your calorie intake in maintenance, it is still invaluable to come back to the system of calorie counting when the need arises. That may be just for a day, or even just to check the calories involved in eating or drinking something new.

• We think that regular weighing is a good idea in maintenance (to be discussed further in slice 50). But we believe that weighing is particularly important if you are going to follow a 'lighter' version of counting and recording calories against a target allowance. You need to be sure that the lighter version is not causing you to start on a slippery slope!

• For the umpteenth time, we see that we are all different, and we need to fine-tune some basic principles, to find what works for each of us. On the face of it, we have both had, and continue to have, similar and successful weight-loss journeys. But in maintenance, Caroline follows a 'slightly light' system of counting and recording calories against a target allowance. Steve, on the other hand, prefers to follow a more informal 'very light' approach. Other people will be different again; everyone has to find their own long-term solution – one that is going to work for them.

# Slice 35

# Understand the changing relationship between calories consumed and burned in maintenance

We explained in slice 9 how, when you are trying to lose weight, it is (for most people) more important to focus on calories consumed than on calories burned. We also explained how, as your weight falls, your calorie allowance falls too, but that you may not *want* to consume fewer and fewer calories. In that case, the option of burning more calories by exercising may become more attractive.

Because you are reading this now, you probably understood what we were saying all those pages back – because if you achieved your target weight, you probably managed to adjust your calorie consumption or burn some more calories (or do both). A great achievement, and one that is going to stand you in good stead as you move into maintenance!

In maintenance, it is still true that your main focus should be on being careful with calories consumed, but the relationship between calories consumed and burned does change slightly, as we will now explain. Let's begin by looking at what is going to make your maintaining job easier and what is going to make it harder.

## Some things that make your maintaining job easier
• You are no longer trying to lose weight, so you can consume a little more or exercise less. But don't go mad – it's not a huge change. We are all different, but, to use ourselves as examples, when we hit target weight, we could ease off by no more than a few hundred calories a day. That's something like an extra sandwich.
• If you have been following this book and not some fad diet, you will have acquired lots of good food habits.

## Some things that make your maintaining job harder
• Every year from your thirties onwards, you naturally lose muscle. This is important because we can think of our muscles as 'little furnaces' that increase our burning of calories even if we are sitting around doing nothing. So as we lose muscle, there are fewer little furnaces, and hence fewer calories burned.

• Losing muscle makes it harder to do physical activity, which means that we tend to do less physical activity as we age, giving us an even lower calorie burn.

• Every year, your metabolic rate slows, so your body burns fewer calories. This is not a huge effect – for every year it's the equivalent of about a pound of body weight. But nevertheless, it is something to be aware of – if you are now in (say) your twentieth year of maintenance, your metabolic rate has been slowing for a long time. You will therefore need to be consuming considerably fewer calories than when you achieved your target weight just to counteract that natural slowing down of your metabolism.

Notice that your maintaining job keeps getting harder and harder as you get older and older. We have just seen that, over time, the effect of your slowing metabolic rate is significant. But add in the other effects – muscle loss and less activity – and we are probably talking about a significant problem of several pounds of body weight every year.

To summarise so far: as your years of maintenance roll on, if you do nothing about it, your muscles will reduce (and your calorie burn will reduce), you may do less physical exercise (and your calorie burn will reduce), and your metabolism will slow down (and, guess what, your calorie burn will reduce). If you are still eating what you always ate, you will therefore put on weight.

You could combat all of this by eating and drinking fewer calories, which may well work. But you may prefer to keep your calories consumed up by boosting your calorie burn and achieving that by increasing your exercise – especially those all-important exercises that build muscle. In any case, exercise is widely beneficial in general health terms, and as we are thinking about the rest of your life, increasing your exercise may be an all-round good idea.

We are aware that this slice is a bit doom-laden. But from here on, it's good news!

**Good news 1.** We just said, 'If you do nothing about it, your muscles will reduce.' That's true, but we *can* do something about it. Muscle can be developed at any time in life. We are not going to attempt to be everyone's personal trainers, but if you are able to exercise (especially doing strength-building exercises), it will benefit your weight maintenance.

We have written slices 23 and 49 to help you – both slices are about increasing your calorie burn, but the second of them concentrates on your calorie burn in maintenance. Incidentally, these are not slices about how to become a fantastic athlete, but rather about how ordinary people (like ourselves) can increase the calories they burn.

**Good news 2.** Even if you are not interested in exercise or not able to exercise, it is entirely possible to counter the effects we have been describing by diet alone. To put it in perspective, consuming just thirty or forty fewer calories every day is enough to counteract the reducing calorie burn we have talked about. It only takes a tiny effort of will to pick up a medium-sized apple rather than a large one – and we have then counteracted that day's reducing calorie burn! So if an opportunity comes our way to save a few calories, we are always open to taking that opportunity.

Frequent weighing and constant vigilance are our friends! If we are careful, it is possible to win the battle with our bodies, which are inconveniently burning fewer and fewer calories every year. Steve is not a naturally boastful sort of guy, but he points out that in the years after he reached his target weight, he won the 'battle with his body'. By being careful with what he ate, even without doing much exercise, his weight carried on drifting down slowly (by about four pounds a year).

Our overall message is that your body's normal calorie burn will reduce as your years of maintenance pass by, but that you can counter this by diet or by burning more calories. We have practical suggestions about both of these in slices 39 and 49.

# Slice 36

# Decide on your approach to
# social eating events in maintenance

There are some aspects of controlling weight that seem to get easier once you get to your target weight and settle into the business of maintaining that weight forever. For example, as we'll see in slice 41, if good shopping habits have become part of your everyday life while losing weight, then they will probably have become automatic, and you will hardly ever think about them in maintenance. Unfortunately, handling social eating events is not like that!

In fact, our experience suggests that difficulties with social eating is one of the main reasons that so many people do not maintain their hard-earned weight loss. We believe that people fail because they think that being in maintenance means they can now enjoy all of their social occasions without being careful about the calories involved and still maintain their weight. To do that might be possible, but we think it's unlikely! So we are now going to look again at some of the difficulties in handling social eating while losing weight, which we identified in slice 10, and then think about how these difficulties can also apply to social eating while maintaining.

We are going to look at this subject largely using two chat times, one of them involving two of Caroline's friends. Gill and Jenn are both long-term dieters and, at the time of the chat, they had lost a fair bit of weight and were maintaining.

### CHAT TIME

CAROLINE: *While you were losing weight, what sort of reactions did you tend to have when you were eating with friends or family but being careful about what you ate?*

GILL: *A mixture really. Some were kind and encouraging and told me how well I was doing.*

JENN: *Yes, I had a mixture too. Many people were nice, although I did have a few too many comments along the lines that one big meal wouldn't hurt or that I was being a spoilsport.*

CAROLINE: I know that you're both maintaining now. Has the negative stuff now eased off?

JENN: To some extent. Although the people who were not very helpful while I was losing weight are probably even worse now!

GILL: Yes, it's the same with me. Many people are really nice, but there are always those who never really accepted why I wanted to lose weight. I have the impression that those people assumed I would 'return to normal' once I got to my target weight.

CAROLINE: They may not realise that, for you, careful eating will be for life. And even if you explain it to them, they may still not be all that sympathetic or accepting. I think I was quite lucky, because by the time I reached my target weight, all of my friends and family seemed to have accepted my changed diet.

JENN: And did they understand that your changed diet was going to be similar when you were a maintainer?

CAROLINE: Generally, yes. But did you find that the snag came more with new people you got to know?

GILL: Definitely yes! Those people had never seen me when I was overweight, and some didn't seem able to visualise me as an overweight person.

JENN. I had this as well. I think some new friends saw my care over what I ate as a little silly – precious, maybe.

GILL: I think that Jenn and I both feel that the problems surrounding social eating in maintenance are certainly there, and need to be handled, but are outweighed by all the positives.

It's important to say that the various difficulties associated with social eating events may not improve over the years. The reason for this was covered in slice 35, in which we saw that as we get older, our metabolic rate slows. So if we don't succeed in the task of burning more calories in exercise, we are going to need to consume fewer calories. And those people who are rather negative about the care we take with our eating will, other things being equal, become slightly more negative with each passing year!

The title of this slice asks you to decide on your approach to social eating events in maintenance. So, after reading several hundred words about how dealing with social eating events in the long term can be difficult, what *should* your approach be? Let's look at another chat time.

## CHAT TIME

*CAROLINE: We had a chat some time ago about our approach to social eating events [that chat was included in slice 10]. I think we found that our social lives were both full ones but notably different from one another. Also that we approached social eating while dieting in different ways too.*

*STEVE: Yes, my approach was rather straightforward – almost brutally straightforward. I told everyone I knew that I was determined to lose a lot of weight, and they were going to have to accept a Steve who was not going to be swayed about what he ate and drank.*

*CAROLINE: And, as I remember, it generally worked fine.*

*STEVE: Yes. Generally. A couple of people were a little put out, but I thought that was acceptable.*

*CAROLINE: My approach was more softly-softly. I was more worried about offending people, so I wasn't quite as blunt as you were. I didn't come out and say I was careful and not to be swayed, but I think they got the message.*

*STEVE: In the end, we both had to have a good think about what sort of activities went on in our social lives, and what sort of relationships we had with the people we knew, and figure out the best way of navigating through it all – while keeping our diets on track.*

*CAROLINE: And it's particularly important to have that good think rather than simply accept that social situations will arise and that you will eat and drink with little or no control. And even more so in maintenance – if you get to target weight, you don't really think about future social events, and you sleepwalk into eating exactly what you feel like eating at every event, then it is easy to put on a lot of weight, and quickly.*

We can't emphasise too much the importance of the subject of social eating. Eating and drinking is a major part of how many people socialise, and being seen as a social animal is, again for many people, fundamental to their sense of self-worth. Add to that the fact that what is eaten and drunk at social events is usually high in calories, and it's unsurprising that many people find it difficult to enjoy their social lives while also controlling their weight. It speaks volumes that a considerable part of our book covers aspects of social eating events.

This slice has set the scene for how to approach social events in maintenance. We will look at specific actions you can take in slice 48.

# Slice 37

# Get support from somebody
# in maintenance

In slice 11 we said that having support – particularly personal support from a 'diet coach' – was important when trying to lose weight. The right diet coach is someone you want to feel accountable to. A diet coach wants to hear about your dieting plans and how you are doing against your plans and is encouraging if things are not going well. They may even put you back on the straight and narrow when you stray. Basically, a diet coach is a friend on a difficult journey. We believe that the usefulness of a diet coach does not finish when you reach your target weight, but that a diet coach is at least as useful in maintenance.

We have already said that in some ways maintenance is even more difficult than losing the weight in the first place. You have learned a lot, especially if you slimmed down in a steady and controlled way, so you probably have some idea of how you need to eat to stay a healthy weight. The snag is that your successful weight loss was probably a fairly short journey, but your maintenance journey stretches out far into the future. If all goes well, it will stretch out forever. After all, if it didn't stretch out forever, that would mean your maintenance would have failed, and that's unthinkable!

If you have successfully lost weight before and then put it back on again, it may have been weeks, months, or even years before you started to put weight back on. But, as happens with many people, you may have started to put weight back on immediately after reaching your target weight. This time needs to be different! And, to help it to be different, it is a good idea that everything – including your diet coach – is in place right from the start.

It seems to us that having the same diet coach in maintenance as when you were losing your weight is ideal, because that person knows you and your weight very well. That is one reason why having a long-term partner as a diet coach can be good. But if, for whatever reason, you need to find a new diet coach, then at least finding one may be an easier task than it was before you started to lose your weight. That's because by the time you are starting maintenance, you will know just what you want from a diet coach, and so which of your friends may be best suited to the role.

You might think that you now need less support than you did during weight loss, but we believe that the opposite is true. Support in maintenance is particularly useful – that's the very time that you need to talk to someone who reminds you what a big deal it has been to lose the weight. Someone who can encourage you not to let it all go to waste now.

Our experience is that we both appreciated our diet coaching almost from the moment we began maintaining, when we hit the wobbles, the uncertainties, and the anxiety about putting the weight back on that many (most? all?) people experience as they begin to maintain.

Once those early difficulties faded, we settled into a routine where we reported our weights to one another at least weekly and where we thought ahead to difficult situations. For example, Caroline gave Steve some suggestions about how he might manage the situation when he was going away on an eleven-day residential course with excellent but calorific food. And when Caroline was having a few months where it was proving difficult to get back on track and her weight had gone up a few pounds, Steve was always supportive but also clear that she had gone outside her acceptable weight band, and he was a little bit challenging about this until she got back on track. So although checking in with your diet coach might not be as frequent as it was when you were losing weight, it's still nice to know that safety net is always there.

The final point we would make about diet coaching leads on from above: Steve 'was a little bit challenging'. We have a diet coaching relationship that is frank and fearless – what we termed 'robust' in slice 11. If Steve thinks Caroline's clothes look a little tight, he says so. If Caroline thinks that Steve is being too slow losing weight after a week away from home, she doesn't hesitate to come right out with it.

We know of other pairs of diet coaches where the relationship is softer-edged and where everything is positive and complimentary. Our impression is that this softer-edged diet coaching is friendly but not as successful at actually controlling weight. Which way you do it really depends on your personal chemistry, but we think that the results of a 'robust' style tend to be a little better than 'softer-edged' – assuming you don't get too upset with one another!

## The Weight Maintenance Manual
### how to achieve and maintain
### your ideal weight

The four parts of The Weight Maintenance Manual are:

Part 1: What you need to understand
so you can lose weight successfully

Part 2: The actions that you need to take
so you can reach your target weight

Part 3: What you need to understand
so you can maintain your target weight forever

Part 4: The actions that you need to take
so you can maintain your target weight forever

# Welcome to

# Part 4

# The actions that
# you need to take
# so you can maintain your
# target weight forever

# Slice 38

# Learn to problem-solve in maintenance

By this point in the book, we hope you have:
• Understood how to lose weight (part 1).
• Learned what you need to do to reach your desired weight loss (part 2).
• Arrived at your target weight (or thereabouts).
• Understood how to maintain your target weight (part 3).

When we started to plan this book, our first thought was that all you would have to do now would be to keep going with everything you did to lose weight. For about ten minutes we were saying to ourselves that part 4 of the book was basically ...

## KEEP AT IT

But after those first ten minutes, we realised that although in an ideal world that's true, it is unfortunately not an ideal world. The difficulty is that although maintaining does have a significant element of 'keep at it', it is clearly not that simple. If it were that simple, nobody would ever regain the weight they lost. And we know that most people *do* regain that weight.

The reason it's not as simple as 'keep at it' is that events in life can get in the way. Some events get in the way after a week or two, some after a month or two, and some after ten years. But however long it is, it's a problem. We are both determined to keep our lost weight off forever, and we want you to do that as well. So in part 4 of the book, we are going to concentrate on what we need to do *in addition to* keeping at it. And the first area we are going to look at is problem-solving.

In slice 12 we talked about problem-solving when losing weight. At the end of that slice we said that, sooner or later, your weight-loss regime will come up against problems. You can use these problems as reasons/excuses to give up the diet for a few days (or longer) or you can learn to problem-solve to find your own solution, and so carry on losing weight. We also went through nine general problem-solving steps that can be applied to all of us. As a brief reminder, these are:

1. Be clear about what your problem is.

2. Think about what solution there may be to your problem.

3. If you see a snag with your solution, don't dismiss it too quickly. Be flexible about how you might do things a little differently, so your solution still works.

4. If you are sure that your solution can't work, don't let yourself get discouraged.

5. Think about another way of solving your problem. Again, don't be quick to reject your solution! How could you adjust it?

6. Don't give up. Keep repeating steps 3, 4, and 5 until you find a solution that you think will work.

7. Once you have a solution that you think might work, try hard to make it work. Be determined. Give it a really good try and, if necessary, adjust your solution as you go along.

8. Despite trying hard to make it work, if your solution clearly won't work, repeat steps 3, 4, and 5 yet again.

9. Be determined that you will find a solution that works for you – keep trying; don't get fed up and give up!

These problem-solving steps are a useful method for tackling difficulties, both in weight loss and in weight maintenance. In fact, problem-solving is one aspect of weight maintenance where if you remember what you did during weight loss, you will go a long way if you 'keep at it' for maintenance. However, the reason 'keep at it' with your problem-solving is not enough on its own may be weight control fatigue. You may remember weight control fatigue from slice 27, where we said that people can start off keeping at it and maintaining well, but then boredom creeps in, things start to drift, and they finally lose control of their weight. Then they get fed up and give up.

Unfortunately, a type of weight control fatigue can afflict one of the most useful tools you have – your ability to problem-solve. You may have come across countless difficulties while losing weight, and you have been creative at getting round those difficulties. But now you are beginning to maintain. You have had enough of being clever with ingredients to save some calories or of figuring out how to avoid drinking too much wine at a family get-together. You just want to give it a rest. And even if you don't think in that way soon after getting to target weight, then you might well think in that way after years of successful maintenance, when problem-solving is just a hazy memory.

If you feel that your interest in problem-solving is indeed on the wane – that you have lost your enthusiasm for sorting out problems to do with body weight – we would like to give you a little pep talk on the subject! The way we see it is that (1) an important part of maintenance success is keeping interested in problem-solving and (2) that keeping interested in problem-solving needs a will to succeed, which springs from being motivated. Let's take those in turn.

**An important part of maintenance success is keeping interested in problem-solving.** We believe that having enough of thinking through your maintenance problems is not just unfortunate, but rather one of the main reasons that maintenance fails and weight piles on again. We have talked to a lot of people who are yo-yo dieters to try to find out *why* it all went wrong after they had lost a lot of weight. They usually (even always) were rather vague about it, but their basic message was that they just couldn't be bothered any more. That's exactly our own experience too. We have never found a study about why maintenance failure happens, but our opinion is that maintenance failure is often (maybe usually) because of a loss of interest in problem-solving.

**Keeping interested in problem-solving needs a will to succeed, which springs from being motivated.** We have just seen that keeping interested in problem-solving is important. But it is also difficult, because you have to maintain that interest for years and years. In order to do *that*, you need the strong desire to control your weight, which is created by being motivated.

The quick summary here is that motivation helps long-term problem-solving, and *that* helps long-term weight maintenance. Obviously, what is called for is a healthy dose of motivation! We suggest, therefore, that if your interest in maintenance problem-solving is flagging, you go back to the slices concerning motivation (3 and then 30), especially concentrating on the idea of the benefits of being at your target weight. We don't think that it's over-dramatic to say that these last few lines are some of the most important in the book!

# Slice 39

# Manage your calories consumed in maintenance

We have said more than once that, having lost weight, you can't go back to consuming what you did before you lost your weight. Well, you *can*, but you will soon be reminded of the truth that

### If you eat what you always ate, you'll weigh what you always weighed

And the *longer* you have maintained at your target weight, the *more* important it is not to go back to doing what you did before you lost your weight. Why? Because you are getting older, metabolism slows with age, and so you don't burn as many calories as you used to.

This is half of an unfortunate double whammy – as maintainers keep maintaining, their calorie burn falls with the passing years. But the other half of the double whammy is that as time goes on, it gets easier and easier for those maintainers to get a bit bored and to lose interest in the subject of weight control. Therefore the risk of gaining weight increases, and that is what happens to an awful lot of maintainers, even after several years of maintenance.

In this slice, we are therefore going to remind ourselves of the key points we made concerning weight loss in slice 13 and see what traps there are in these key points for a successful maintainer – and how the traps can be avoided.

We suggested that you set yourself a daily allowance of calories you are going to consume. There is probably not too much difficulty here – as a successful calorie-counting dieter, you probably have a good idea of how many calories you need to consume to keep your weight steady, so 'keep at it' will be helpful. You just need to remember that for every year you age, your calorie burn reduces. The effect is not much in a single year, but after several years, it becomes substantial.

We said that in a calorie-counting system, it is a good idea to consume what you want within your calorie allowance but to be careful not to fool yourself by under-recording calories consumed. These are still perfectly valid thoughts in maintenance, but the particular enemy in maintenance is weight control fatigue. As a reminder, one sort of weight control fatigue is where you eat more high-calorie foods (or simply more food) – often without really noticing what you are doing. Or you might notice what you are doing but fail to include the foods in your daily calorie counting. Of course, if you are totally focused and self-disciplined, such things never happen, but here in the real world they happen a lot. And the longer that time goes on, the more likely you are to fall prey to weight control fatigue.

You can get some protection from weight control fatigue by following the suggestion we made in slice 13 to keep a running total of how many calories you have consumed. However, there is often excitement when losing weight, and that excitement may have been sustained over (at least compared to the many years of maintenance) the fairly short time between starting your diet and reaching your target weight. You may have remained keen to measure everything and calculate a running total of calories. Maintenance, however, is different because you are now faced with doing those things forever. Some people (Caroline is an example) happily do that, but others (such as Steve) don't want to count and record calories permanently. Caroline needed to interrogate Steve a little on this subject.

### CHAT TIME

*CAROLINE: I can accept that you don't count and record calories any more, and it certainly seems to be working, but why is it working?*

*STEVE: I think what I do is a reasonable second best. After several years of maintaining, I have a good idea of what I should and should not eat in order to maintain my weight, so I don't usually keep a daily running total. But I do so when it really matters.*

*CAROLINE: I obviously need to prise this out of you! So, when does it 'really matter'?*

*STEVE: It really matters when I see that I have clearly miscalculated, my weight has increased, and I have not managed to bring it down again to where I want it to be. That doesn't happen often, but when it does, I go back to basics and keep a daily running total. And I make sure that total is low enough for me to lose weight.*

*CAROLINE: Yes, I can see that. Your system does depend a lot on weighing yourself quite often, to get an early warning of when your weight is increasing. And weighing is also important to make sure that you are managing to lose the weight. But I suppose that is just the same as it was when you were 'dieting'.*

So we do suggest that maintainers either
• measure their calories against a daily calorie allowance every day, or
• measure their calories against a daily calorie allowance, if and when the scales tell them that their weight has increased and they are having difficulty bringing their weight down again.

In slice 13 we also warned against resisting the temptation to 'take out an overdraft'. What we meant by that phrase was overeating now while promising yourself that you would clear the overdraft at some time in the future. Our warning was because in the real world, paying back such a calorie overdraft rarely happens. In maintenance, our warning is even louder because we may have an added difficulty – it might be getting easier and easier to lose interest in the subject of weight control. In that case, it becomes *even harder* to clear that calorie overdraft – the next day or ever.

We also talked about fad diets. They often don't work when you are losing weight. And if they didn't work then, you might think that there's no reason for them to work now you are maintaining. However, the reason you might be mellowing towards fad diets when in maintenance is the old story – boredom (just another type of weight control fatigue). You could put up with restricting your calories in the modest amount of time that you were successfully losing weight, but now you are maintaining and, as we often say, that's forever. We think, therefore, that it's a good idea to keep up your interest by eating in a new and interesting way – by being more adventurous with what you cook and how you cook it while keeping calories reasonably low. We both think that the other's cooking is getting more and more interesting while tasting better and still delivering fewer calories. We are not professional cooks, merely enthusiasts who are trying to keep our diets interesting. If we can do it, you can! Experiment a bit!

But if you don't want to work on developing your range of ingredients and your cooking, but instead you really, really, really want to try that new eating regime where you only eat after noon, and even then you just eat pork chops and passion fruit (or any other fad diet), then give it a go. It's your life. Maybe it will suit you, and maybe it will work well for you. What we suggest, though, is that you put a limit on the regime – maybe you are only going to try it for a month or maybe you are going to stop if you put on seven pounds. But set a limit, stick to it, and go back to your tried-and-tested weight-loss diet in order to return to your target weight! Please – do this for us! Imagine what a tragedy it would be if all of that hard work to lose weight was ruined by persisting with an eating regime that wasn't working.

We also strongly recommend that you keep going with SPCs – small permanent changes to your pre-weight-loss diet, which we also discussed in slice 13. Maintenance can be hindered for various reasons, many of them linked to (1) calorie burn reducing with age and (2) just getting slightly bored with the whole business of being careful about what you eat. Constantly thinking of new SPCs is a way of fighting back against these problems. Our friend Zoe had something to say about this.

### CHAT TIME

*ZOE: I know you two are very keen on SPCs, and I have made some of them, and I can see why they are a good idea …*

*CAROLINE and STEVE: We can see a 'but' coming up soon!*

*ZOE: Mmm, but … how can they be useful in maintenance? You often say that we need to find new SPCs, and that's difficult enough. But to do that for maintenance will be impossible, won't it? Maintenance is going to go on for a very long time, so won't we just run out of ideas?*

*STEVE: Always the one with the tricky questions!*

*ZOE: I bet you've got an answer, haven't you?*

*STEVE: Yes indeed! Maybe the best approach is for Caroline and me to give you some examples of recent SPCs we've come up with. We have several years of inventing SPCs under our belts, but we still have some fresh and new ones.*

*CAROLINE: I've got one to do with cooking – I have always tended to taste food a lot while I'm cooking, so my SPC was to cut right back on doing that. A few calories saved. Steve, another!*

*STEVE: Even though I now make low-calorie curries from scratch, we have always had a spoonful of commercial chutney or pickle to go with it. I stopped doing that, because the commercial chutney is packed with sugar and the commercial pickle contains a lot of oil. Caroline, over to you!*

*CAROLINE: I have experimented with low-alcohol beer, but then I noticed that one of them (the nicest one, as it happens) was much less calorific than the others. So I now often drink a beer that is low-alcohol and low-calorie. Steve!*

*STEVE: The same for me with low-alcohol wine. I just put up with the fact that it doesn't taste too good. Caroline, your turn!*

*ZOE: OK, OK, enough! I'm convinced you can keep dreaming up new SPCs. What a pair of clever-clogs!*

*CAROLINE: Seriously, it's not a matter of being clever. It's just like a game – spotting these small calorie savings that are going to battle against the small calorie effects of slowing metabolism and possible waning interest in the whole business of dieting. It can be a fun game, and it's a game that's well worth playing – because playing the game helps you to keep at your target weight forever.*

Now for a final and important point. As we often say, maintenance is going to be for a long time. During such a long time, different people may come into your life or leave it. Especially if they join or leave your *household*, there may be dramatic changes to your eating and drinking patterns. Imagine, for example, the possible changes to your eating regime if you acquired a new partner, complete with children. Imagine further (this was our example way back in slice 1) if your new partner did not *want* you to be slim and the children left chocolate biscuits lying around as if to tempt you. This is just one example – our relationships, and our lives in general, are often complex and ever-changing. It is simply impossible for this (or any other) book to suggest how you can maintain your target weight in the face of changes in your life in your decades of maintenance. But we hope that you will at least have the possibility of finding a solution by looking again at slices 12 and 38 concerning problem-solving.

In this slice, we have looked at some of the possible problems in controlling calories consumed that a maintainer can encounter. Many of these problems involve weight control fatigue, which we believe is one of the biggest problems (if not the biggest problem) that a maintainer can face. We will come across the subject of weight control fatigue several more times in the book!

# Slice 40

## Change what you eat and change how you cook in maintenance

We saw in slice 14 that if you want to change your eating habits, there are only two possibilities. Those possibilities are (1) to eat the same foods that you have always eaten, but less of them, and (2) eat different foods. We would guess that, as a successful dieter, your weight loss was helped by doing both of those.

Here in part 4 of the book, we have already said that it is not good to arrive at your target weight, breathe a sigh of relief, and go back to doing exactly what you did when you put all your weight on. So it is pretty obvious that in maintenance, you need to carry on in a similar way to when you were losing weight. Or, as we often say, 'keep at it'.

But 'carry on in a similar way' doesn't mean identically, and therefore 'keep at it' needs some further thinking in order to achieve successful maintenance. So here are two developments of our advice in slice 14, which we hope you find useful as you set off into that 'forever' that is maintenance.

### Keep your food varied and interesting

As we said above, losing weight probably involved both eating less of the foods you had always eaten *and* eating some new foods too. As you move into maintenance, you may think about going back to 'normal eating' by reversing what you did when losing weight. In other words, by increasing those foods that you used to eat and reducing the new foods that you introduced. This could work, but it's not something we would recommend, for two reasons.

• In general, going back to anything like your pre-weight-loss diet 'normal eating' feels to us like you are moving back to 'eating what you always ate'. And that, of course, feels like you are moving back to 'weighing what you always weighed'. Maybe that's not true for you. Maybe you are able to go back to something like your pre-weight-loss diet 'normal eating', but you have learned all about portion control of those foods you used to eat, so you will be able to keep a good grip on your maintenance weight. Maybe. But it seems a bit risky to us. We prefer to have a maintenance eating regime that has a lot of new foods in it, sending a signal to ourselves that we are in a new part of our lives.

• A problem of increasing old foods and reducing new ones is that your eating regime approach becomes one of controlling forever your consumption of those 'old foods' – the very foods that made you overweight in the first place. Those foods were probably moreish, containing a lot of fat or sugar (or both). Your task in maintenance would therefore become one of limiting your consumption of moreish foods – foods where you have a history of being *unable* to limit them. To us, this seems *more* than a bit risky.

We therefore think it would be easier and more successful in maintenance to keep eating a modest quantity of foods you always used to eat, but also to keep eating foods that were new to you while losing weight. But having said all of that, it is obviously up to you. If you are convinced that in maintenance you can go back to a restricted version of what you used to eat, and hence manage to keep your weight stable for many years, then go for it. You might succeed. All we would ask is that you keep weighing yourself and take seriously what the scales are telling you. If the scales are telling you that your weight is gradually going up, that may be the time to change your approach before it's too late and you end up back where you started. Which would be a huge disappointment.

There is something else to say on this subject, and it's quite good news. Let's see some chat time.

### CHAT TIME

CAROLINE: *It's possible for tastes to change. Humans are programmed to like familiar foods, so if you eat less of something, it gradually becomes less familiar to you – and then, amazingly, you start to lose interest in it. That happened to you, didn't it?*

STEVE: *Yes, it did, and it's been useful for maintaining my weight. In an earlier chat time [in slice 14] I said that while I was losing weight I actually stopped eating quite a lot of high-calorie foods altogether. Although that's not a recommended technique, I found that when I got to my target weight, I had lost interest in some of those foods, and nowadays I eat them only rarely.*

CAROLINE: *Which foods were they?*

STEVE: *Pasta was one – I used to eat a lot of it, but nowadays it might be once a year.*

CAROLINE: *In a way, pasta is quite easy to lose interest in. Apologies to pasta lovers, but it doesn't have a particularly fascinating flavour. What about foods that contain lots of fat, sugar, or salt – notorious problem foods such as chocolate, crisps, or cheese?*

STEVE: *It's a mixture, really, with no obvious pattern. I tried to give up cheese but never lost interest in it and didn't quite manage to give it up, although I did manage to cut down my consumption.*

CAROLINE: *Maybe, in that case, you were still eating so much cheese that the taste of it never became unfamiliar?*

STEVE: *Possibly. I certainly had no such trouble with chocolate and crisps – I completely gave them up and later found that I had lost interest in them.*

CAROLINE: *Wow – lost interest in chocolate! I don't think many people could honestly say that!*

STEVE: *Yes, I know it's unusual, but it may have been partly because I was never that attached to chocolate anyway. But what about you? Did you lose interest in anything while you were losing weight?*

CAROLINE: *Not really, because my weight-loss diet was largely one of eating less of what I used to eat before the start of my diet. So I was never likely to lose interest in certain foods because I kept on eating them while losing weight – although I didn't eat them in big quantities. Clotted cream is the one exception I can think of.*

STEVE: *Clotted cream! An amazingly calorific food. It's not difficult to help yourself to a modest-looking portion and later realise that it was a 500-calorie dose!*

CAROLINE: *Yes. My love of cream (especially clotted cream) was legendary among my family and friends. But somehow, when losing weight, I managed to stay away from clotted cream for a while. And, what's more, a year after giving up clotted cream, I was persuaded to have some as a 'treat', and I was shocked to find that my taste had changed completely. It wasn't a treat, I didn't enjoy it, and I wouldn't be trying it again!*

*STEVE: It shows again, and for the umpteenth time, that we are all different, and that there are many different ways of succeeding with a diet (and many different ways of failing, of course!). So the summary is that some people can lose their taste for calorific foods and if they do, it is useful in maintenance.*

*CAROLINE: So that's good news. But I'm afraid there is some bad news to go with it. The bad news is that, whether or not you lost your taste for high-calorie foods, that loss may not be permanent.*

*STEVE: Unfortunately, you're right. I think we've done well as maintainers – certainly between us we have a fair few years of maintenance under our belts. But we still get occasional urges to eat too much of certain things.*

*CAROLINE: Yes. I have always had rather a bad relationship with biscuits, and since I lost my weight and have been maintaining, it has been better. But better does not mean perfect! Occasionally, life can be going along fine, but then there's a slight upset and biscuits have strangely disappeared from in front of me and there are crumbs around my mouth.*

*STEVE: Yes, I know just what you mean. But for me it's bread – especially when there is cheese around as well. And, even worse, now I am several years into maintenance, I occasionally find myself eating and enjoying foods for which I was certain I had lost the taste – a taste never to be regained (so I thought!).*

*CAROLINE: Is there any particular trigger that you've noticed?*

*STEVE: Not an obvious one, no.*

*CAROLINE: Mmmm, annoying, isn't it? And what's more, I*

*don't think I have ever met a successful maintainer who has said anything different. We all, as the years go by, find that there is a small but annoying tendency to slip back into eating too much of foods we thought we had finally gained control over.*

*STEVE: It looks like we are all going to have to wait for some amazing scientific discovery. Until then, we need to exercise constant vigilance and realise when we are eating 'occasional foods' so often that they have become 'frequent foods'.*

*CAROLINE: And if an occasional food changes to a frequent food, you will need to decide whether to keep eating it so often. If you do, you may need to have a rethink about the full range of foods that you are eating.*

So we have not yet entirely lost our taste for foods that could easily undermine our weight maintenance; maybe we never will lose our taste for them. But we think it is important to keep varying our food and how we cook it so it continues to be interesting and enjoyable – and keeps at bay what we *don't* want to make a habit of. We are always on the look-out for interesting new ingredients and for interesting new recipes, and we intend to keep doing that.

### Watch out for weight control fatigue
So much for looking at unwelcome trends in *which* foods you are eating. Now we move on to unwelcome trends in *how much* you are eating. This is another example of weight control fatigue where, you may remember, your eating regime goes along just fine but, bit by bit, you lose your grip and your weight starts to increase.

The type of weight control fatigue we are referring to here is when the portions you ate when losing weight begin to grow in size. This is clearly a problem if it's cheesecake and probably *not* a problem if it's lettuce. But it's the in-between foods, which you may not even think about much, that need special attention. We saw Steve's perfect example in slice 25, when his 40-gram dieting portion of porridge had drifted up to 60 grams, and that represents about a half-stone weight gain in a year.

The drifting of portion sizes is easily done in maintenance – if not in a few weeks, then maybe in a few months or years. And if the drifting portions are not just in one food but in several, it is easy to miss that something is wrong until your favourite clothes no longer fit.

Once more, the message is 'constant vigilance'. Keep paying attention to *how much* you are eating – not just the obvious high-calorie foods, but *anything* that is capable of making you overweight again. That includes nutritious *and* calorific foods, discussed in slice 13!

It's absolutely fitting, in a slice about watching what you eat in maintenance, to finish by mentioning those kitchen scales that were your friend when you were losing weight – keep them in a cupboard close at hand, ready for action!

# Slice 41

# Shopping habits in maintenance

We said in slice 15 that shopping in the right way is at the heart of eating well, and eating well helps you to lose weight. We also gave you ideas about how to plan your shopping and what to do in the shop itself. In brief, we suggested:

• Don't go shopping without having a plan of what you are going to be eating.
• Make a shopping list.
• Buy only what is on your shopping list.
• Buy only the amounts that are on your shopping list.

Shopping is something that you probably do often, possibly even every day. So if you lost your weight over many months and used those ideas about how to shop, you will have used those ideas a lot – maybe hundreds of times. With any luck, many of those good shopping habits will have become part of your everyday life and, in maintenance, you now do them automatically. For example, you wouldn't now dream of going round a supermarket without a shopping list (would you?!).

Unfortunately, as the years of maintenance go by, those automatic shopping habits can become *less* automatic. They may even stop entirely. You may rightly suspect this is another example of weight control fatigue.

### CHAT TIME

*CAROLINE: We both think we are pretty good at shopping, and that that was one of the reasons we managed to lose the weight we did and have managed to keep it off. But we never pretend that we are perfect, and I know we have examples of where we had good habits while losing weight, but the habits loosened when maintaining.*

*STEVE: Indeed! One example, while I was dieting, was when I decided to limit any ready meals I had to 250 calories per portion. The choice of such meals was not huge, but they were not bad at all. I was perfectly happy to eat them, and it was just part of my shopping routine to put only the under-250-*

*calorie meals in the trolley. That carried on into maintenance for at least a year.*

*CAROLINE: I sense some dramatic twist is coming.*

*STEVE: You're right. One day I saw a nice-looking meal, but it was 350 calories. I bought one 'just to try it', and it was really good. So I started to buy that meal regularly as well. And then – well, I was buying a 350-calorie meal anyway, and there were other nice-looking 350-calorie meals on the same shelf, so I started buying those too.*

*CAROLINE: Of course, everything you did was perfectly reasonable – after all, as a maintainer, you could eat more than when you were losing weight. But if you gradually let go of those good habits you acquired while losing weight, you will eventually get to a point where you are consuming so many calories that you start to put on weight.*

*STEVE: It's a good example of weight control fatigue. What about you?*

*CAROLINE: When I was dieting, I learned very well not to even go down the supermarket aisle where they put the chocolate biscuits. But over time I started to wander down 'just to see what was new' and then, a little later, I bought a packet of some of those new biscuits 'just to see what they were like'. You can probably see that I was beginning to live more and more dangerously. Once more, it's weight control fatigue.*

*STEVE: And this is the way weight control fatigue usually happens – bit by bit, with each bit looking harmless enough. The odd chocolate biscuit or an extra 100 calories on a meal is nothing to get excited about. On their own, they are, indeed, harmless enough. But the problem, as we have both realised more than once, is where those slippery slopes lead to!*

What we would like to emphasise from everything above is that as the years of maintenance continue, it becomes more and more likely that weight control fatigue will interrupt those good shopping habits you acquired while losing weight. Especially because, in maintenance, you will be able to consume more calories without weight gain than you could while trying to lose weight. That can easily lead to feeling overly relaxed about the whole business of shopping (and even maintaining in general).

The issue, therefore, is what you can *do* about this shopping-related weight control fatigue. The most obvious thing to do is make use of the book in your hand – go back to slice 15 and make sure that you are still doing what we suggested there. In other words, have a plan of what you will be eating, make a shopping list, and buy only what is on that list.

Remember also that habits, other than totally ingrained ones, need some effort to remember and some effort to keep doing. So every time you go shopping, pay attention to what you're buying – and we're not just talking about obviously high-calorie foods, but anything that is capable of making you overweight again. That includes those nutritious *and* calorific foods, which we have mentioned before (in slice 13, for example).

# Slice 42

# Enjoy your food and eat without guilt for the rest of your life

We saw in slice 16 that there are difficulties in trying to completely cut out enjoyable (often high-calorie) foods as part of a weight-loss diet. We also looked at how it is possible to continue to lose weight while still enjoying – without guilt – such 'non-diet foods'. That's much better than telling yourself that you can never again have foods that you love.

If, during weight loss, you *did* follow our advice in slice 16 and you learned how to continue enjoying 'non-diet foods', then we think you will find maintenance of your weight loss easier. We like the idea of keeping *some* room in your life for high-calorie foods that you really enjoy. But the challenge in maintenance is *not* to start to eat *unrestricted amounts of everything* you didn't have much of when you were dieting! It's true that there is a little more 'wriggle room' in maintenance for eating some higher-calorie foods, but you need to be careful – there is probably not as much wriggle room as you hoped. Remember that if you go back to eating *exactly* as you were eating before you dieted, you will end up as heavy as you were before you dieted.

On the other hand, if you *did not* follow our advice in slice 16 and, in fact, you completely cut out some higher-calorie foods that you love – and intend to keep them out of your eating regime permanently – then we think you will find maintenance of your weight loss hard going. You *may* find that you have lost all interest in those foods you gave up. But if you are still keen on them, you will be faced with the difficult task of resisting them forever. You may then decide to re-read slice 16 and see whether you want to follow our advice after all – the section 'It's possible to eat anything you like and still stay on your diet' is the one you need.

There is another snag in maintenance, which we discussed in slice 35: as we age, our muscles reduce and our metabolism slows down. If (like many people) we do not put in considerable and regular physical effort, the result is that we *burn fewer calories*. On the other hand, if (again, like many people) we experience weight control fatigue, the result is that we *consume more calories*. This is an unfortunate double whammy, because burning fewer calories and consuming more calories is an obvious recipe for weight gain. So, again, we need to be careful not to eat *too many* of those higher-calorie foods in maintenance.

Having talked about challenges and snags, maintenance does include some good news – tastes can and do change. There are probably foods you didn't like as a child which you came to like as an adult. And there may well be foods you didn't like at the start of your diet which you like today.

Hopefully, you will keep discovering new foods that are lower in calories *and* that you really like eating. You might like to refer back to slice 14 about changing what you eat and how you cook it. The slice contains a lot of information about introducing more interesting and enjoyable foods into your diet.

So, to summarise this slice, in order to enjoy your food for the rest of your life:
• Keep at it – keep doing what you learned in slice 16 while you were losing weight, but ...
• be careful not to eat too many more high-calorie foods, and keep being careful as the years pass, because your body burns fewer and fewer calories as it ages.

Finally, we're going to introduce another idea, which applies to this slice and also to most slices in the remainder of the book. The idea is *Steve and Caroline's Maintenance Review*. It is a simple but effective idea for combating weight control fatigue – a regular check for maintainers to confirm that their maintenance is on track. Most of us want maintenance to be a less onerous occupation than losing weight, and so our regular review is straightforward. It's as follows:

### Steve and Caroline's Maintenance Review

1. Occasionally have a week of keeping an exact running total of how many calories you have consumed. In other words, go back to the basics of controlling calories consumed (see slice 13).

2. Regularly weigh yourself (see slice 24).

3. Regularly check whether you are straying from your long-term goal (see slice 33). If your long-term goal is simply a body weight, this will be the same as number 2.

221

We are not going to tell you exactly how often is 'occasionally' or 'regularly'. We have come far enough in the book together for you not to need such detailed instructions! To give you an idea, we think that it's reasonable, every three months, to (1) go back to basics on calorie counting and (2) weigh yourself and check where you are against your long-term goal. That should help you to keep on track and give you good early warning if you are beginning to slip. Both of us do the review regularly, and we believe that it is an important part of our maintenance success.

# Slice 43

## Don't use food as a reward in maintenance

In slice 17 we discussed using food as a reward – in other words, automatically reaching for food when we feel pleased with ourselves. We explained why, although it may seem perfectly reasonable to reward yourself with food, in fact it is not a good idea. Not even when you can 'afford' the calories. We finished the slice with the cheery thought that, on the whole, people who reward themselves with food are overweight. And those who don't – aren't!

What's more, rewarding yourself with food was not a good idea when you were losing weight and it's still not a good idea now you are maintaining your weight. Although if you are reading this now, having successfully lost weight, we think that it is unlikely that you are still *frequently* rewarding yourself with food. But you might still be doing it if you found a good way to reward yourself with food and you still lost weight. On the basis of 'if it ain't broke, don't fix it', you could just carry on.

You may, however, not want to carry on. Instead you might want to kick the food-as-a-reward habit. In that case, you could do worse than go back to slice 17, re-read it, and have another go.

Even if you feel that you are no longer tempted to link good and bad events in your life with food (or drink) rewards, you need to be careful in maintenance. As we have said frequently elsewhere, for most people successful maintenance lasts a lot longer than the successful weight loss before it. There is plenty of time in maintenance to return to old habits, even those habits you thought you had broken years ago.

We ourselves are not immune from slipping back to the old habit of rewarding ourselves with food. Our celebrations, following something we are pleased to have done, occasionally involve old favourites such as biscuits, wine, cheese, and whisky (not all at the same time!). What we do, however, is to recognise that we *did* reward ourselves with food. That awareness helps us to avoid doing the same thing the next time. We believe that's the reason we now usually think of rewards in non-food and non-drink terms.

This slice is another strongly 'keep at it' slice, with the added advice to keep track of how your maintenance is doing to make sure that things are not slipping. This time the risk is that a slip might be happening because of a growing tendency to reward yourself with food. Another clear case of the usefulness of *Steve and Caroline's Maintenance Review* (see the previous slice).

# Slice 44

# Change the way you deal with surplus food in maintenance

In slice 18, back when we were looking at weight loss, we discussed how you can get good at *not* eating surplus food, and we saw why that is a useful skill to have. So what do we need to pay special attention to once we get to maintenance? That depends on whether you really *did* get good at not eating surplus food while losing weight. We are going to look at that by using the biggest chat group in our book – not only the two of us but also three friends we had previously talked to about dieting.

## *CHAT TIME*

*STEVE: Hello, welcome everyone! Pete and Hannah, let me start with you two – when you were losing weight, did you get to grips with the idea of not eating surplus food?*

*PETE: Yes, I did. I got quite good at doing it and over my year of dieting, I threw away a fair bit of stuff. But, to be honest, I always thought it was odd to bin perfectly good food, and in maintenance I'm going to return to acting more normally!*

*HANNAH: You did better than I did. I thought it was odd from the very beginning and never even thought about binning food.*

*CAROLINE: But you both got to your target weights recently, didn't you?*

*PETE and HANNAH: Yes.*

*CAROLINE: So, big congratulations! What about you, Charlotte?*

*CHARLOTTE: I followed the advice of Caroline and Steve, and I got good at not eating surplus food. In the end I was pretty comfortable doing it, and I've been carrying on with the same ideas in maintenance.*

PETE: But don't you get people criticising you for throwing food away?

STEVE: *I think the secret to this* [and this is what we wrote in slice 18] *is that there are ways of avoiding eating surplus food other than throwing the food away.*

CAROLINE: *That's true. Literally throwing away surplus food is pretty much the last resort – there is nearly always something else you can do with it. You can freeze it, give it to others (for example, family, friends, neighbours, food banks, or your builders), or put it out for your local wildlife.*

HANNAH: *That makes sense. But if you do end up giving food to your friends and family, it still seems slightly weird to me. Didn't it ever bother you?*

CAROLINE: *I suppose it depends on your friends and family. I think that the people I know learned years ago that I would rather send surplus food to the bin or to somebody else's house than consume it myself. Maybe for a short time they thought it was slightly weird, but they soon got the idea, and they stopped trying to persuade me to consume surplus foods. That made it all easier.*

CHARLOTTE: *It was the same for me. Everyone is now completely relaxed if I give them a goody bag when they go home after eating at my place.*

STEVE: *And me. There is always the likelihood, in our years of maintenance, that we will all get to know new people – family, friends, or work colleagues – who will not understand that giving away food (or even throwing it away) is fine. They may come out with the same friendly (but weight-increasing) thoughts that we heard years ago – such as 'Oh, go on, finish that dessert, it'll only go to waste.'*

CAROLINE: *That's been my experience, but then I just have to gently explain once again why I do not want to be a human dustbin. It does need some tact, but I owe it to myself to do it, to maintain my weight where I want it to be. I have found, and I know that Steve has too, that I've got better and better at not*

226

*eating surplus food (or drink for that matter), and that includes these occasional little social challenges.*

*CHARLOTTE: And I've certainly found that the good habits in this area have become easier and easier to retain. I'm sure it'll work out fine for Pete and Hannah as well.*

That chat time all seems very positive, but we do know that dealing with surplus food is not always simple. Whatever sensible points were made above (and in slice 18), a lot of people have a strong and instinctive resistance to giving dinner guests surplus food to take home or – perhaps especially – throwing food away. We do both of those things, and quite happily too, but we do know that it's not for everyone.

Of course, you are not obliged to follow every piece of advice we offer! You will be able to maintain your weight by following our advice on some matters but not on others. If ideas such as getting rid of surplus food do not appeal to you, then it may not be a disaster if you keep eating the surpluses. But it's always a good idea to do as many things as possible to support your weight loss and weight maintenance ambitions, and that becomes more and more important. Why? It's because as the years of maintenance roll on, changes in your life make your weight control more difficult. For example, (1) you need fewer calories because of ageing, (2) other good habits may begin to slip, (3) you may find yourself in different family or social situations.

If you find, therefore, that your weight is starting to increase beyond what you are comfortable with and you *are* still regularly eating your food surpluses, you can always go back to slice 18 and see whether our ideas about dealing with surpluses now appeal to you. Those ideas may give you another useful tool to control your weight.

# Slice 45

## Learn how to manage your hunger in maintenance

In slice 19, we looked at how our bodies make us hungry as a reaction to our eating less and losing weight. We looked at how to manage our hunger and we saw that being able to manage hunger is fundamental to dieting success. In fact, we reckon that if you are reading this now, at your target weight, you must have got pretty good at that key dieting task of hunger management. So if that is you, and on the basis of 'if it ain't broke don't fix it', just continue with what you are doing – this is another of those 'keep at it' slices.

But. So often there is a but! Maintaining your weight forever is a long-term project, and life does not always run along straight tracks. Changes may occur because of new friends, family, illness, and so on, and your eating habits may start to alter. Maybe, for example, you have a new partner who can eat anything and not gain weight (so far!), and that may influence what you want to eat. If you *do* start to change your eating habits, then changes that make you feel hungry are something to take seriously. Rediscovering what it is like to live with frequent hunger is a dangerous path that carries a real risk of regaining some or all of your lost weight.

A much better idea than regaining your lost weight is to go back to eating what you did while dieting (and maybe re-reading slice 19, about managing hunger while losing weight, would help). In addition, we do have some more thoughts that might help you to manage your hunger. We could have included them in slice 19, but we thought there was quite enough to absorb in that slice already. Maybe these new thoughts will give you some fresh ideas if you are a maintainer who is beginning to struggle.

### Manage hunger before it happens by eating foods that stop you getting hungry

If you can do this, then your hunger may never develop. What these foods are that stop you getting hungry varies from person to person. Caroline, for example, finds that vegetables and salad work well. Steve finds that both porridge and salad stop him getting hungry for hours. Other people do not find that at all – for example, they swear by high-protein foods to keep them feeling full.

There is no one-size-fits-all answer, but we recommend that you experiment with various foods to see if you can find something that works for you. It is well worth spending some time on this because if you *can* find a food that is a hunger-stopper for you, then you have a useful weight-loss and weight-maintenance tool for your whole life. We even suggest that the benefits are so valuable that it is worth trying foods that you are not particularly fond of – you could *grow* to be fond of them!

**Manage hunger before it happens by eating at certain times**
Some people find that eating at certain times stops them from feeling hungry, or at least it slows down the development of their hunger. Those 'certain times' are, once more, personal things. For example, some people find a decent breakfast fills them up until lunchtime, but other people find they are peckish just an hour after eating it. And some people are not hungry in the evening after eating their last meal of the day in the late afternoon. Others would be starving all evening if they did that, and they need to have dinner at eight o'clock. Again, it's not one size fits all, and you'll need to experiment with different meal times.

Of course, you really hit the jackpot if you find foods that reduce your hunger *and* also times of meals that reduce your hunger. Steve is a good example: he has a big bowl of porridge at eight a.m. and is still not hungry at lunchtime, and for lunch he has a big bowl of salad and is then not usually peckish until at least eight p.m. He just tried lots of different combinations of foods and mealtimes and, in the end, was lucky. But you can't get lucky unless you try things!

**Manage hunger if it does happen**
We used to think that if we felt hunger coming on (before lunch, for example), it was a good idea to have a 'little something' early to tide us over until lunch itself. Generally, we don't think that worked well. What happened was that we ate that little something and then we ate the lunch we were going to have anyway. So we just ended up eating more calories than we had intended.

Now, when we feel hunger coming on, we just tell ourselves, 'Don't worry, lunch will be in just half an hour.' It's simple and effective. But if we are still tempted to have a 'little something', we remind ourselves what we said in slice 19 – that feeling hungry is (1) something that we don't need to cave in to, (2) not dangerous, (3) something we can put up with it until our next meal, and (4) easy to confuse with being thirsty – drinking a big glass of water can make those hunger pangs disappear!

# Slice 46

# Handle emotional eating
# in maintenance

Your task in maintenance seems straightforward. You succeeded in losing weight, which is a considerable achievement, so now 'all' you need to do is keep doing the same – forever. But in the case of emotional eating, keeping doing the same is difficult, because your life is unlikely to stay exactly the same forever. Emotional changes may happen, possibly leading to overeating.

In slice 31, we explained three aspects of emotional eating that were particularly important to understand in maintenance. Those aspects boil down to three questions:
• Even if you overcame your emotional eating, is it returning?
• For 'spur-of-the-moment' emotional eaters, are your emotional triggers changing?
• For longstanding emotional eaters, are deeply ingrained habits resurfacing?

The essence of slice 46 is to consider the answers to these questions and look at what you can do about them.

### Even if you overcame your emotional eating, is it returning?
On the face of it, dealing with emotional eating in maintenance may not seem like a big problem – after all, you managed to find a way to tackle your emotional eating before, so you can do it again. And that may be true – except you can only start to do it again *if you actually know that your emotional eating has returned.*

That is the heart of the problem. If you use the bathroom scales to weigh yourself regularly, you can see that you are gaining weight, and you can then return to good weight-losing eating habits. But, unfortunately, there are no 'emotional scales' that can tell you that your emotional eating is increasing and that it is time to do something about it. But there is something we mentioned in slice 31 that you *can* use to assess whether you are eating emotionally or not – ask yourself two questions about the last time you overate:
• Were you content, involved in what you were doing, or with pleasant people? If so, that does not sound like emotional eating.

• Were you bored, lonely, sad, angry, frustrated, scared, or any combination? If so, that does sound like emotional eating.

We think it is a good idea for maintainers to have regular reviews at which they ask themselves those questions – perhaps you can put regular dates in your diary to remind yourself? It may seem odd to make something so formal out of the subject of emotions, but you can use your answers to decide whether your emotional eating is increasing and to do something about it as soon as possible, before you put on a lot of weight and get fed up and give up.

Once you know that your emotional eating *has* returned, the actions to take to address the problem are exactly the same as those we discussed in slice 20, when we covered how to handle emotional eating during weight loss. So please refer to slice 20 but, as a quick reminder, those actions were to describe the emotion, to delay eating, to distract yourself, to eat something else that's lower in calories, and to notice how you feel when you eat something in response to an emotion.

### For 'spur-of-the-moment' emotional eaters, are your emotional triggers changing?

Spur-of-the-moment emotional eating is a difficult part of maintenance. If, while losing weight, you managed to find out which emotions triggered your eating, that was a hard job, and well done. But in the many, many years of maintenance, most people's lives change, and those triggering emotions can change as a result – sometimes without warning and sometimes quite dramatically. So it is useful to keep thinking about which emotions trigger the occasions when you overeat.

We suggest that part of your regular reviews (above) could be to think about whether you are experiencing *new* emotional triggers and, if so, what those triggers are. Having done that, you can again refer to slice 20, because what to do about changing emotional triggers is the same as returning emotional eating, discussed above.

### For longstanding emotional eaters, are deeply ingrained habits resurfacing?

During weight loss, longstanding emotional eaters can sometimes manage the difficult task of consciously changing a deeply ingrained habit. But in the long years of maintenance, there is the possibility that the deeply ingrained habit can resurface, despite seeming to have disappeared. It is important to know this resurfacing is happening, and the quicker the better – the longer a deeply ingrained habit is re-established, the harder it will be to shift.

We have three thoughts about how to tackle deeply ingrained habits that may re-establish themselves in maintenance:

• Be aware that such re-establishing is possible and (a bit of a theme in this slice) aim to identify it as early as possible. Yet again, a regular review of how you are doing – backed up by entries in your diary – is a good idea. Constant vigilance is key!

• If you did manage to achieve success with one or more deeply ingrained habits while losing weight, you now have a big advantage if they start to re-establish themselves in maintenance. That is because you now know what those deeply ingrained habits were and what you did to tackle them. So you have a good idea of what to do this time.

• You have a further advantage when dealing with re-establishment of deeply ingrained habits – deeply ingrained habits were laid down a long time ago, often in childhood. So whatever those habits are, it is unlikely that new ones are appearing. Maintainers will therefore tend to be dealing with the same few issues, even though they might be difficult ones. This is in contrast to the issues facing spur-of-the-moment emotional eaters, whose problems can be brand new as life throws something different and unexpected at them.

Finally in this slice, we would like to repeat what we have said about emotional eating elsewhere in the book. It is a difficult area, so although you may make good progress on your own, the involvement of health professionals or counsellors may be useful or even necessary. But even if it takes time to get the support you need to make changes, don't get fed up and give up while you are waiting. Simply having read our thoughts on emotional eating will have made you more aware of the subject, and that alone may help you to make significant progress.

# Slice 47

# Handle cravings in maintenance

In slice 21, we went through some ideas about how to manage cravings. If you became good at managing cravings while you were losing weight, this was probably one of the many successes that helped you to get to your healthy weight. However, by their very nature, cravings are hard to banish forever, and so you may find that they are still an issue in maintenance. Crisp cravings were certainly still a problem for Zoe, and the following is the discussion that she had with Caroline on the subject.

*CHAT TIME*

*CAROLINE: Well done on reaching your target weight. I hope you are very pleased with yourself!*

*ZOE: I am, mostly! But I am still having some cravings for crisps – cravings that I give into. That isn't helpful. I'm worried it might be a weak spot in my maintenance, and I don't want to put the weight back on.*

*CAROLINE: Did you use the approach we discussed?*

*ZOE: Describing, delaying, and distracting?* [We covered this in slice 21.] *Yes. Sometimes it was helpful and other times less so.*

*CAROLINE: If it was ever helpful, that's a good start – and one approach would be to continue practising until it is helpful more often.*

*ZOE: I feel like I've been doing that forever – since I started my diet!*

*CAROLINE: OK, how many packets of crisps do you eat?*

*ZOE: It could be three or four packets a day.*

*CAROLINE: And how do they get into the house?*

ZOE: I buy them.

CAROLINE: Do you buy them because you think something dreadful will happen to you if you have a crisp craving and don't satisfy it?

ZOE: I think you're teasing me! No, of course not!

CAROLINE: So is it because you think that you have cracked the crisp craving issue?

ZOE: Sadly not! Oh ... then I shouldn't be buying them at all?

CAROLINE: If they are not in the house, you are much less likely to eat them!

ZOE: Does that mean I can never have crisps again? I thought it wasn't a good idea to try and cut things out altogether.

CAROLINE: There certainly are problems with cutting foods out. Have you thought about buying just one packet of crisps at a time?

ZOE: Mmm, that might help. The nearest shop is a long way away, and I probably wouldn't want to go out for another packet just after eating one.

CAROLINE: Or, if that doesn't work, you could try going 'cold turkey', despite the problems with cutting foods out entirely.

ZOE: What sort of problems are they?

CAROLINE: Cutting out can make cravings stronger or make people feel deprived and more likely to give up on their weight control overall. These problems can be even worse if they cut out a lot of foods that they used to like.

ZOE: That's not good, but maybe I could at least try crisp 'cold turkey'.

CAROLINE: Yes, you could. As in many other aspects of dieting and maintenance, everybody is different. For example, some people cannot cut foods out of their diets without feeling *deprived, while others (Steve, for example) can completely cut foods out for years without a problem. So 'cold turkey' could work for you. You never know.*

*ZOE: OK, thanks. I think, to begin with, I'll try buying just one packet at a time. But if that doesn't work, I'll try crisp 'cold turkey'. I'm not keen on the idea, but I really don't want to put the weight back on. I'll give it a go.*

Zoe was very aware that her cravings were still likely to cause a problem to her goal of keeping the weight off forever. Not everyone is so alert to the dangers, however. It is worth checking from time to time whether foods you had stopped eating or were eating very infrequently are creeping back into your daily diet. If your weight is remaining stable, then you are probably managing it well. But if your weight is rising, a good place to start trimming back is on foods you *know* you can cut down because you have before. And now is the time to do so again!

Please don't underestimate the problems of cravings in maintenance. We said at the start of this slice that cravings are hard to banish forever, and while we were writing this book we had a surprising illustration of how hard it can be – close to home.

### CHAT TIME

*STEVE: I know you use me as an example of somebody who can completely cut foods out of his diet.*

*CAROLINE: Yes, I do – it's true, isn't it?*

*STEVE: It was true. In fact, cutting food out was one of the most successful elements of my weight loss. I know that it is not a widely recommended technique, but I was careful not to cut out essential nutrients. So I cut out quite a list of foods, including oil, pasta, rice, pastry, cake, chocolate, and biscuits.*

*CAROLINE: And in several years of maintenance, you have kept most of these foods off the menu.*

*STEVE: I do have some of them very occasionally. But I have just lost the taste for some foods, especially cake, biscuits, and chocolate. For a long, long time – in dieting and in maintenance – not one morsel of cake, biscuits, or chocolate passed my lips. And it was easy.*

*CAROLINE: I sense an 'until' is coming.*

*STEVE: Until I was in a café a few weeks ago. I had some tea and, for some strange reason, it seemed like a good idea to have a huge piece of coffee cake. The first piece of cake I had had for several years. I don't even particularly like coffee cake!*

*CAROLINE: Oh well, these one-offs don't do any harm.*

*STEVE: If only! For some weeks after that I had quite a few cakes and biscuits on various occasions, and I could see that they were adding a lot of unwanted calories to my daily intake.*

*CAROLINE: That is odd: you have a reputation as someone who has remarkable willpower when it comes to what he eats.*

*STEVE: Mmm. Anyway, there it is. The good news is that I started to gain a little weight and I didn't have too much trouble in taking cake and biscuits back off the menu. That did the trick, and my weight returned to where I wanted it to be.*

We thought it was worth putting Steve's 'confession' in this book. He is something of an expert dieter and an expert maintainer, so if – after years of cutting out certain foods – Steve succumbed to cravings for some of those foods, then cravings in maintenance certainly seem to be a foe to be taken seriously.

# Slice 48

# Handle social eating events
# in maintenance

We hope that, in slice 22, you learned something useful about handling social eating events during weight loss and that that knowledge helped you to reach your target weight. That should make it easier for you to get to grips with the slice you are now reading, because it is another slice where 'keep at it' applies.

Generally, your life should be a little easier in maintenance because you will have a little more calorie 'wriggle room'. But the problem with that, which we will discuss, is that once you allow yourself some more calorie flexibility, you need to know when to *stop* allowing yourself calorie flexibility.

In this slice, we are going to use similar headings to those we used in slice 22 and discuss the extent to which 'keep at it' applies and the extent to which we now need to make some adjustments.

### Be wary of forgetting your calories entirely
We said in slice 22 that, when losing weight, it's important to be wary of forgetting your calories entirely where social eating events are involved. Now you are maintaining, there is no harm at all in *keeping* interested in calorie consumption during social eating, but perhaps it is not essential – *as long as your maintenance is going well*. But – and it's a big 'but' – you do need to know whether or not your maintenance *is* going well.

If you have an active social life but you have lost contact with the world of calorie counting, then it is useful (in our view, essential) to get clear confirmation that your maintenance is going well – by stepping on the scales. And that weighing has to be frequent enough, so any weight gain it reveals is not too great. You do *not* want to get fed up and give up!

### Plan for single events
We looked, in slice 22, at the idea of saving some calories in the days before an event such as a night out and, if necessary, saving some in the days following the event too. We were only thinking of a single event, where any weight gain would be small, and so this 'penny-pinching' of calories would often work without resorting to any drastic daily calorie reduction.

237

Once your maintenance is well-established, we think that such fine control of body weight for a single event is probably unnecessary. There is a good case for going to the event and enjoying the food on offer without guilt. After a few months of maintenance, we both found that we had acquired enough maintaining ideas and habits to recover a small weight increase caused by a single event without too much effort.

But you need to be careful not to fall into the trap of going to such events too often, especially if you are not taking much care over the calories you are consuming. This is an easy trap to fall into because if you allow yourself to do it once, it makes it easier to do it again and again. In the end, you may be going to so many nice events that you are not really maintaining any more, and you are slipping back to the disastrous situation of eating the way you did before your weight-loss diet even started. Of course, you will pick this up soon enough (as we said a little earlier) if you are weighing yourself regularly. If you are not weighing yourself regularly, there is a danger of gaining a lot of weight, so you get fed up and give up.

## Plan for a series of events

We are now talking about a series of events, such as a weekend of celebrations or a two-week cruise. In slice 22, we looked at the idea of losing weight before (and probably after) a long social event where we were sure that we would gain considerable weight. Perhaps surprisingly, our conclusion was that, for most people, the risk of eating badly and getting fed up was too high. And we suggested that it was best to accept any weight gain and also to accept that you might put back the date of hitting your target weight.

We left slice 22 saying that compensating for such things as holiday weight gains was different once you got to maintenance and that we would look at that in slice 48 – so here we are! Let's cover this one with some chat time involving Steve and Orlagh, a friend who had been maintaining for a couple of years.

### CHAT TIME

*ORLAGH: I've heard you talk about the idea of losing weight before going on holiday as 'Ann's idea'. I know that Ann's your wife, but how is it her idea?*

*STEVE: Good question! While losing weight, I had always tried to save some calories in advance of a big, calorie-laden meal. But quite often I didn't manage that and ended up the day after the meal with a weight gain that I had to try to get rid of.*

ORLAGH: *That seems normal enough.*

STEVE: *Yes, and it was OK. But then I got to my target weight and started to maintain, but a few weeks later Ann and I were going on holiday for ten days. I seriously overdid it and returned home nine pounds heavier.* [We mentioned this story in slice 29.]

ORLAGH: *Oh dear. But you were a good dieter by then, so I suppose you lost it again OK?*

STEVE: *In the end, yes. But it took two months, and I was worried that I might lose my grip and end up regaining all the weight I had lost. I moaned about it constantly, and Ann was getting really fed up with me.*

ORLAGH: *No wonder. So come on, tell me about Ann's idea.*

STEVE: *OK. In fact it's very simple – Ann said that rather than putting on weight and getting worried about it, if I was going to a longer 'special event' and I thought it was likely I would put weight on, then I should try hard to lose that weight before the special event, not after.*

ORLAGH: *So if I weigh ten stone before Christmas and I always stay with the family for five days at Christmas (and always seem to put on five pounds), then I should slim down to 9 st 9 lb before I go. So I will lose those five pounds before Christmas, and when I return I haven't gained any weight.*

STEVE: *Exactly. And it's not too difficult for any maintainer to have a reasonable guess at how much they might put on. Even if you're not a regular calorie counter, it is more than likely that you have been through it all before – whether at Christmas time or during a two-week holiday.*

ORLAGH: *Right, I can see this. Ann's lose-it-first technique might look a bit daunting, but it's much better than doing nothing, going to the event, feeling bad, risking giving up, then fighting to get back to where you started before the event.*

*STEVE: It's much better. And, instead, you feel good because you are doing something positive to prepare for your special event, you have a great time, then you return no heavier than before your preparations started. And don't worry if your guess at what you will put on isn't quite right. If you guess three pounds, lose that three pounds, but only put on two pounds, then, as a maintainer, you will find it easy to ease off slightly and get back to your target weight.*

*ORLAGH: And on the other hand, if you guess three pounds, lose that three pounds, but then put on four pounds, then that's still good. Because if you hadn't used Ann's idea, you would now be four pounds heavier, with a slightly increased inclination to get fed up and give up. Either way, maintainers win, and there are not many things in life you can say that about – thanks, Ann!*

Ann's idea seems such a winner, you may be wondering why we are discussing it for maintainers *only*. We talked about this in slice 22, so maybe you would like to go back and re-read it. In a nutshell, it's because many dieters need to reduce their calorie intake to quite a low level in order to lose weight at all, and so reducing their intake even more to compensate for the effects of something major (like a holiday) would be difficult. It might encourage unhealthy undereating and getting seriously fed up. But maintainers have more calories to play with – they have the ability to reduce calories so that they can lose a significant amount of weight.

Having said all of that, Ann's idea is not some magic solution, and it needs motivation and determination like everything else to do with weight control. Steve has used it successfully, but people who we have spoken to about it are not always immediately taken with it. There seems to be a deep-seated belief that the natural way of dealing with some major calorie-consuming event, such as a holiday, is to throw caution to the wind first, then be 'punished' for it afterwards. But we like Ann's idea a lot, and it's worked for us, so it's here in the book – try it and see what you think!

## Choose carefully what you eat at social events
In slice 22, we based our thoughts about choosing what to eat at social events on the powerful saying 'You don't have control over what you are offered, but you always have control over what you eat.' Then we spent time looking at how that saying applied to bring-and-share events and

to holidays. This is a clear case of 'keep at it' in maintenance. It's true that in maintenance, you have some more calories to play with. But if, while losing weight, you acquired the useful habit of choosing from what is offered at social events (rather than eating and drinking on a sort of automatic pilot), then that is all to the good.

## Enjoy what you eat

There is no point in a social eating event if you are not enjoying what you are eating. We said it when talking about weight loss (see slice 22), and we are now saying it when talking about weight maintenance. For us, this is an essential 'keep at it'.

We both feel that an important part of our success at losing weight was that we retained our love of eating and drinking and never felt guilty about what we were enjoying. This was so important to us that we devoted a whole slice to it (slice 16). In maintenance it continues to be important – how could it not be? Otherwise, we would be faced with having a bad relationship with food and souring our social activities for the rest of our lives, which would be unthinkable.

## Social pressures

It may seem obvious that if you learned how to deal with the pressures to eat and drink in social situations while losing weight, then you would have no trouble dealing with those pressures when maintaining.

Unfortunately – and you may remember this from slice 36 – life does not always run so smoothly. People you are in regular contact with may expect that you will 'behave more normally' in your social life now that you have reached your target weight. You will probably also acquire new friends and relatives who may also wonder why you don't 'behave more normally'. Being seen as a social animal is important to very many people, and so they want to behave according to the norm. But as more 'normal behaviour' in social events often involves high-calorie eating and drinking, the socially active maintainer can find it difficult to keep control of their weight in the long term. What is the solution to this?

The answer is largely about communication. When talking about dieting in slice 22, we covered the subject of social pressures by means of some chat time with Zoe. She went on to slim down to her target weight, and we talked to her again after she had been maintaining for a few months.

## CHAT TIME

CAROLINE: So, Zoe, welcome back! And very well done for getting down to your target weight.

ZOE: Thanks. And I'm managing to maintain more or less at that target weight. But I've got to say that the help you gave me with social pressures hasn't always worked out.

CAROLINE: Why? What's gone wrong?

ZOE: Well it has been OK with some people – I explained it all to them, that I needed to stick with being careful. Some people were nice about it and some were not quite so nice. But while I was losing weight, it was generally OK, and I avoided too many calorie mishaps.

CAROLINE: And that's fine. There can't be many dieters who have been perfect every single step of the way.

ZOE: Yes, but it has not always worked out so well since I have been maintaining. Even I have to admit that I am now reasonably slim, and the sort of comment I now hear a lot from my family and friends is that I don't need to diet anymore, so why can't I eat and drink just what everyone else is having? It's making me feel something of an outcast.

STEVE: I understand that. For me, it's not been too bad – during weight loss I handled my social eating problems by flatly telling people I was on a diet and that was that. It was a bit brutal, but it was absolutely clear what I meant, and most people accepted it. In maintenance I just use the same approach.

ZOE: But what do you say when people point out that you are no longer on a diet, so you don't need to be careful anymore?

STEVE: I just tell them the honest truth.

CAROLINE: Yes, I've heard him do this several times. He says that in a way he is still on a (modest) weight-reduction diet, *because from time to time he does overdo things and puts some weight on, so he will probably have to be careful forever.*

*STEVE: And it works. Because when I do overdo it a little on social occasions, people often advise me to be careful! They have learned that from me telling them so often!*

*ZOE: So what you are saying is that if I explain to people that I will always have to watch my weight, they will accept that and be nice about it?*

*CAROLINE: You can never be certain how people are going to react, but Steve and I have found that it often works. And especially if you explain why you will always have to watch your weight.*

*STEVE: Most people I've met have never come across the idea that you will have to be careful forever if you want to keep at your target weight forever (and that that means that you can't eat much more than you did while losing weight). They find it surprising and interesting, they usually understand it, and they are then on your side and happily accept your little dietary 'foibles'.*

In the same way as when you were losing weight, however carefully you think about these issues and however well you communicate with people, sooner or later you will be in a situation where the social pressure to eat something that you would rather *not* eat is very hard to resist. In that case, we think that it is perfectly fine not to attempt all the explanations but just eat it and enjoy it without guilt (remember Caroline's 'tartiflette moment' from slice 22?). As a maintainer, you have some calorie 'wriggle room', and hopefully you have all the weight-loss skills you need – you can lose that little bit of weight that you put on because of that irresistible pressure.

The only snag we can see with this 'just eat it' approach is if somebody says something to you like 'Oh, go on, you know you want that big slice of chocolate cake,' and you reply, 'No, I won't, thanks,' but your social circle has seen you eat chocolate cake before. In that circumstance, they start to think that you don't really mean it, they keep on pressing you, and you end up always saying yes. This is a steep and slippery slope, with a high risk that before too long you are no longer thinking like a maintainer and your weight starts to rise. So it is important to be consistently firm about what you will or will not eat.

## A final thought on this slice

The general theme of this slice (and related slices 10, 22, and 36) is that it is extremely important for both dieters and maintainers to deal with the difficulties of social eating events.

We have seen that it *is* possible to adjust calorie intake so that social eating does not derail weight loss or weight maintenance. But this is a big ask. We certainly found it so on the many occasions in our lives when we (1) became overweight, (2) did not adjust our calorie intake enough, and (3) saw our weight continue to creep up. We therefore have a history of failing. It is only recently that we think (hope!) that we have finally cracked it.

It's hard. But there is something quite exciting shining in the distance. There is a theory that there are only a very few people who have 'slim genes'. Most people who seem to be 'naturally slim' do not have 'slim genes' at all – they are merely people who, without any big drama, adjust their calories from day to day. If they have a big meal, they simply consume less food on the following day to balance things out.

We find that really encouraging. It could be that if we all keep working away at keeping our weight on an even keel by adjusting our calories before and after an excess (for example, in some social setting), then, in the end, it will become an instinctive habit. Certainly, we both feel that if we can change ourselves from seriously overweight people to effortless maintainers, then that will be one of the great achievements of our lives.

# Slice 49

# Keep up your calories burned in maintenance

As time passes, weight control fatigue makes it easier and easier for maintainers to become slightly bored and to lose interest in the subject of weight control. This causes two problems: a tendency to *consume more calories* (which we looked at in slice 39) and a tendency to *burn fewer calories* (which we are now going to look at).

There are three main reasons that we burn fewer calories in maintenance.

• Our metabolism naturally slows, and that means that it burns fewer calories (also discussed in slice 39).

• It becomes easier to get bored with exercising (in the same way as becoming bored with watching our food intake).

• Our bodies tend to get less and less able to do the exercise.

The first two may be clear already, but the third may need some explanation. You may have read it thinking that it does not apply to you because although you are getting older, you are pretty athletic and are still able to do a lot of exercise. If so, that is fantastic news. But you are exceptional – from simple observation, it seems that most people do not include much exercise in their lives as they pass into middle age. And people who continue burning more and more calories right up until their dying day are so rare that they are featured on the national news!

It's tough, but that is just how life pans out. It gets harder and harder to do exercise, but it's good to keep doing it, and it's good to be ambitious about what you can do. Also, exercise is useful and enjoyable, and we now have some thoughts about how to do more of it.

In slice 23, we suggested that it is a good idea to measure the exercise that you do. We gave the example of getting yourself a cheap pedometer if walking is your thing. Once you can measure the exercise, then you can record it somewhere. There's no need for expensive technology – a piece of paper is fine. Then once you can record it, you can set yourself targets.

Equipped with measuring, recording, and targets, you have good control over your exercise. Perhaps you can spot when your exercising is gradually reducing, so you can decide to reverse that trend. Or perhaps you can gradually increase your targets. Whatever you *do* want to do, measuring, recording, and targets will make it much easier.

In the same way as liking a variety of foods, it is good to be able to take advantage of different sorts of exercise. Apart from simply getting bored doing the same thing all the time, variety is useful in case you are no longer able to do one type of exercise. This is particularly useful as we age because the body has a nasty habit of breaking down, and even a minor problem can interfere with your favourite exercise. For example, a minor injury to a knee can stop you from walking for several weeks (or even months), while arthritis in your foot can stop longer walks for good. Walking may no longer be an option, so you might, for example, swap to swimming. In that case, measuring, recording, and targets will still serve you well, even though what you use to do the measuring will be different.

We both have some experience of extending our own range of exercise, so let's see a little chat time.

### CHAT TIME

*STEVE: I seem to remember that you used to be a swimmer.*

*CAROLINE: I swam regularly while losing weight. But almost as soon as I started to maintain, I began to find that it was becoming harder to get in enough swimming to have much effect on my calorie burn. The reasons were simply because of my work and because of new opening times at the local pool.*

*STEVE: Did you then swap over to some other exercise?*

*CAROLINE: Probably not as quickly as I should have done. There was no other exercise I liked that immediately came to mind, but then I thought about walking. I've never been very keen on walking, but I began to think of it more as lovely walks rather than exercise, and that did the trick. Since then, walks have become my main exercise. Walking is your exercise too, isn't it?*

*STEVE: For a long time, yes. In fact, I built up from very few steps at the start of my weight loss to a daily average of about 12,000. But recently, although I still enjoy walking, I have found my daily steps have decreased a lot. That's because walking takes a long time, and pressure of work has meant that I have very little time available.*

*CAROLINE: Simply not having time is quite a problem.*

*STEVE: Yes, but I think I've found a way round it, which is to start doing more intensive exercise. I could do with that anyway because I need to build up some muscle, so I am starting muscle-strengthening exercises, and they burn the same calories as my walking used to – but in a shorter time.*

What this chat time illustrates is that there are different sorts of exercise, even for people (like ourselves) who are no longer in the first flush of youth. So, especially in that very long time that is weight maintenance, it is useful to be prepared to swap from one form of exercise to another. If one sort of exercise becomes more difficult to do, try something different – there is an enjoyable type of calorie-burning exercise out there for *you*!

We have already mentioned in this book the idea of SPCs (small permanent changes). It may be worth reminding yourself of the examples of exercise SPCs we gave in slice 23. SPCs are good during weight loss but even better during maintenance, where that triple whammy of lower calorie burn, boredom, and reducing physical ability is always working against you. You'll need SPCs in order to fight back and keep burning as many calories as you can.

Remember that although SPCs are *small* permanent changes, small changes are *still* worth identifying and building into your everyday life. Something as simple as hiding the TV remote and getting out of your chair to change channel will burn extra calories, and we have even worked it out for you – it will burn off about a pound in a year! And that is just one tiny SPC – find fourteen tiny changes and you will lose a stone!

Another positive thought is that – although we are not suggesting it's common – there are people who never took any exercise in their lives, decided to give it a go as part of trying to lose weight, and liked it so much that they took it up seriously. They hit their target weight, just kept on with their exercise, and, probably not a coincidence, they became successful maintainers. Some are quite young, but not all – a couple we heard of were in their sixties. It may need some careful selection of appropriate exercise (see above), but it is possible to continue developing fitness into middle age and beyond. Which is a nice thought for all of us.

Finally, it's important not to run away with the idea that burning more and more calories is some easy option. It is a difficult task for most of us, and so gaining control over calories consumed is always going to be important.

# Slice 50

# Weigh yourself regularly and
# record it in maintenance

In slice 33, we introduced the idea of creating flexibility in long-term weight goals by setting an acceptable weight band – rather than a fixed weight. This is what we did, and our weights have consequently bobbed up and down from time to time, and so have the weights of other successful maintainers. It is fine for your weight to fluctuate within a band, and even the occasional big slip is OK. But you need to be careful – if the slip gets too big, it may become a real problem. You might slip so much that the situation seems irrecoverable, and you may get fed up and give up. There are plenty of people who have maintained a large weight loss for years and then find that, somehow, the weight 'just crept on again'. We don't want that to happen to us, and we don't want that to happen to you either!

Our main suggestion in this slice is, although you may stray from some of the good techniques you used to lose weight, *please make sure that you continue to weigh yourself regularly*. In fact, we think that this is one of our most important suggestions in the whole book.

Weighing and recording in the long term is roughly a matter of continuing to do what you did while losing weight – another case of 'keep at it'. That will become clear, because we are now going to take the five important questions dieters ask about weighing while they are losing weight (which we discussed in slice 24). Then we are simply going to add 'in the long term' to the end of each question and answer those questions as well. Here goes:

**Why is it important to weigh regularly in the long term?**
Many people hope to be able to stop weighing when they arrive at their target weight. Some people believe it is no longer necessary. Some people don't want to carry on weighing because it is associated in their minds with the restrictions of dieting. Others have heard that there is something odd or unhealthy about weighing regularly.

We see it differently. Only by regular weighing will you be able to tell whether your weight is staying within your chosen acceptable weight band. If you watch your weight carefully, you will be able to see if you are slipping and take action quickly. And the quicker you take action, the easier it will be to reverse a weight gain by returning to those good habits that helped you to lose weight.

There is another bonus to regular weighing once you are at the weight you want to be – it is a satisfying feeling to see that your weight is where it should be! You can be pleased with yourself and proud of what you have achieved. At last, after all that dieting, stepping on the scales can be fun and rewarding.

And there is yet another bonus. Weighing yourself regularly in maintenance and seeing the weight in the band you have chosen helps you see yourself as someone who is in control of their weight. The more you see yourself like this, the easier it becomes to make the choices that help you *stay* in control of your weight.

However, we have heard more than once (and we referred to this in slice 30) that it was motivating – while losing weight – to see the scales regularly confirming the good news. *But* that the motivation is weaker in maintenance, when good news consists of the *same news* again and again and again! Steve talked about this with Eleanor.

### CHAT TIME

ELEANOR: *I've been maintaining for a year now, but I don't get the same satisfaction of jumping on the scales every week that I used to. For example, my last four weighings have been 10st 2lb, 10st 3lb, 10st 2lb, 10st 2lb. It's good news, but not very exciting!*

STEVE: *It's a good start that you are at least carrying on with weighing yourself regularly, but I do know what you mean.*

ELEANOR: *Caroline tells me that you have your own system, which helps to keep you interested in maintenance. What's the secret?*

STEVE: *I wouldn't really call it a secret. But what I did do was realise that there were things that were going to help (or hinder) my maintenance that I could conveniently measure every day.*

ELEANOR: *Great! I do like measuring!*

STEVE: *That's good. Some people are not interested in measurements, so this probably won't help them much. But it was good for me. My measurements, other than my weight, were about my steps and about my alcohol consumption – I had the strong impression that too few steps and too much alcohol tended to push my weight up.*

*ELEANOR: Yes, that probably applies to me too. So what is a good level for me?*

*STEVE: That's impossible for me to say, because it depends on the individual. But I thought that my own 'good levels' on any day were (1) my weight was between 12st 6lb and 12st 11lb, (2) I had done 6,000 steps on the previous day, and (3) my alcohol units for the previous seven days were within government guidelines. And as a little bit of fun, if all of those were satisfied when I got out of bed, I gave three cheers, to the embarrassment of my wife! So I called these my Three Maintenance Cheers.*

*ELEANOR: I like the sound of this, although I usually swim rather than do many steps.*

*STEVE: Exactly. The Three Maintenance Cheers is completely flexible – you can alter what you want to measure and alter your 'good levels' as suits you. In fact, I change my own from time to time – my steps used to be 5,000, but I thought I would challenge myself a little more. And, incidentally, I like to keep my Three Maintenance Cheers tough for me – most days I fail on at least one of the three measures, so it's quite an event to get my Three Maintenance Cheers (to my wife's relief!).*

## How often should I weigh myself in the long term?
We both weigh daily, but anything between daily and weekly seems to work best for most people. Don't just take it from us! The National Weight Control Registry is a continuing long-term study of over 10,000 people who have lost weight and kept it off for a long time. Something that most of these successful maintainers of weight loss have in common is regular and frequent weighing – somewhere between daily and weekly. Join the gang!

## Do I really have to record every single weight in the long term?
Many people find that actually *recording* their weight helps keep them honest. Recording weight is also an encouragement, which is useful

because the rewards of years and years of maintenance are not as obvious as the rewards of a relatively brief period of successful weight loss. Keeping a close eye on your ability to keep your weight within a narrow band, even if you are simply writing your readings down on a piece of paper, gives a sense of satisfaction – and that can help keep you motivated.

So, to answer the question, it may not be absolutely essential to record your regular weighings, but we both do it, and we find it a useful tool to help us keep our weight under control.

**What do changes in my weight really mean in the long term?**
Maintainers can be concerned that their weight keeps going up and down when they want to be able to maintain a *stable* weight. In fact, if you want the scales to show (let's say) 10 st 5 lb every single time you get on them, you will almost certainly be disappointed. That's because there are many things that can affect a particular weighing (see slice 25 for details).

The near impossibility of keeping to a particular weight is exactly why we both adopted acceptable weight bands, which we talked about in slice 33. The question then becomes how wide can the band be? In other words, what weight can you go to before you need to do something about it? We did look at the subject of acceptable weight bands in a chat time in slice 33, but here are some other thoughts on the subject, taken from the same conversation.

### CHAT TIME

*STEVE: We've both been maintaining for quite a long time. Do you think that we are now both comfortable that our weights still go up and down?*

*CAROLINE: Reasonably comfortable, yes. But it's still important to set a target weight, with a band of how much it is OK to go higher or lower. Because if you just vaguely think 'I'll stay around 10 st 5 lb', then what do you do if your weight goes to 10 st 7 lb or 10 st 10 lb?*

*STEVE: And without some firm limit on how high your weight should go, it's all too easy to think, 'I've put on another couple of pounds; that's not such a problem.' And then it's easy to think in the same way when you've put on another couple of pounds. And so on, and so on.*

252

*CAROLINE: And all the time, your clothes might still fit fairly well, and you can kid yourself that nothing much has changed. Even though it may well be that you have been in this situation before (maybe often, if you are a confirmed yo-yo dieter). So – NO! You do not want to let this weight-loss victory slip out of your grasp!*

*STEVE: It's important to set an acceptable weight band. My band is from five pounds higher than my target weight down to five pounds lower than my target weight.*

*CAROLINE: And mine is three pounds higher than my target weight down to four pounds lower than my target weight. It's a personal choice, but the acceptable weight band shouldn't be too big. We like to think of this acceptable band as yo-yo dieting, but on a short string!*

If our weight goes up towards the top of our band, we take action to bring it back down again. And occasionally one of us will find our weight approaching the bottom of our band – honestly, it can happen, especially if you have embedded lots of small permanent changes (see slice 13) into your life. In that case we have the pleasant challenge of eating richer foods or a bit more of the foods that we now eat less frequently – but we don't do this for long!

### I just really hate weighing myself – do I have to in the long term?
Earlier in this slice, we suggested more than once that maintainers should weigh themselves regularly. So it's not surprising that we feel the answer to the question above is 'Yes, you do have to weigh yourself in the long term', for the reasons we have discussed. However, we know of a few long-term maintainers who maintain not by regular weighing but by how their clothes fit – so it can be done. But we think it is a risky approach.

The main danger we see is that for many items of clothing, you can put on a lot of weight before they become obviously too small. Remember how long it took to lose enough weight to go down a clothes size? Well, it is the same in reverse! That means you will have been slipping into unhelpful eating habits for some weeks before you realise that your clothes no longer fit. And that assumes that you are being scrupulously honest with yourself.

If you are being *less* than honest with yourself, it is all too easy to wear a different pair of trousers – a pair that is more comfortable. Or you could tell yourself that something must have shrunk in the wash. Then a few more weeks of overeating have set in before you realise that even your 'loosest' trousers are no longer wearable. By this time, you will have got out of many of your good habits and may have regained your taste for fatty and sweet foods.

Any or all of those things mean that getting back on track and losing weight again will be as hard as it was to start the weight-loss diet in the first place. Which is extraordinarily bad news! And all that anguish could have been avoided by weighing regularly.

So we are going to make a heartfelt repetition here: yes, we think that maintainers really do have to keep weighing themselves. Of course, if people absolutely don't want to, that is entirely up to them, but we do think that it is a dangerous approach with a high risk of dieting failure.

We know that we are being unusually insistent about the benefits of weighing in maintenance, and you may have guessed why. It is because both of us have a long history of doing what we are now urging you not to do! We have been seriously overweight, then slimmed down, then stopped weighing, then become seriously overweight again. Often. We are sure that the reason we finally broke this vicious circle is that we realised the importance of regular weighing in maintenance. Anyway, that's enough nagging – let's go on to the next slice!

# Slice 51

# Don't be discouraged if you haven't lost as much as you 'should have' in maintenance

In slice 25, we saw that if you are generally creating calorie deficits, you will also generally be losing weight. But what you can't do is create a calorie deficit in, say, a particular few days and then be sure of seeing a corresponding weight loss in those same few days. Our message is that there are just too many complications of the human body to make such a corresponding loss certain. People who do *not* realise that are almost certain to get fed up and give up. So we think that if you are reading this now, having achieved your target weight, then it is likely that you absorbed our message.

You may therefore be thinking *what is there to say here?* You're maintaining, so why should you be interested in a calorie deficit not corresponding to a weight loss? That's a good question, but it *does* become important for most maintainers, because most maintainers do not stay at exactly the same weight, day after day or year after year. Their weight moves around a little – for example, it may go up after Christmas or after a holiday. When a weight gain happens, *that's* when they want to lose that surplus weight, so they create a calorie deficit in order to lose the surplus. The same might happen to you.

In theory, everything is fine. When you were losing weight, you learned (maybe by reading slice 25) not to expect a calorie deficit to show on the scales immediately. But now, in maintenance, your patience may be tested as never before – you may find that trying to lose weight can be harder than it was during your original diet! That may be because:

• It might be some years since you got down to your target weight, and your body burns fewer and fewer calories as it gets older, so it's harder to create a calorie deficit.

• If you have been maintaining for a long time, you may have stopped counting your calories carefully (or at all), and you may be eating more than you think you are. This is classic weight control fatigue, which we have talked about elsewhere in the book (in slice 25, for example).

We are both typical maintainers, in that our weight bobbles around quite a bit, meaning we have to follow a weight-loss diet occasionally to bring us back to our target weight. Often it is painless, but sometimes the weight loss is disappointing, possibly because of weight control fatigue. And that is the danger time. In the same way as when we were slimming down to our target weights, the risk is that we (or anybody) can get that old feeling of unfairness, get fed up and give up.

If that thought of giving up even flickers through your head, we suggest that you first revisit slice 3, which discusses motivation. Then go back to slice 25, concerning getting back on track during weight loss – if that slice helped you before, it will help you again! We also strongly recommend going back to whatever system you used to lose weight (for example, calorie counting and recording). Use that system and stick with it strictly for as long as it takes to return to your maintenance target weight. As we said above, we have had to do this ourselves occasionally and, so far, it has always worked.

# Slice 52

# What to do to get back on track
# after straying in maintenance

By this point in the book, we hope that you have lost weight and that you are now maintaining. We hope our book has given you an understanding of how to lose weight and maintain your weight loss and that you have benefitted from our specific advice about what to do to achieve your aims.

Unfortunately, it is perfectly possible that something has gone wrong and that you are now unhappy with your weight. Please don't beat yourself up about it – life is complicated, and things can happen to derail all of us. The purpose of the slice you are now reading is to give you a safety net just before we leave you. It contains our suggestions about what to do to get back on track when you have strayed too much from your maintenance target weight.

In slice 33 (which you may like to read again), we talked about what your target weight should be in maintenance, and we said that it was a good idea to be a little flexible. For example, rather than setting a fixed weight, you may want to set an acceptable weight band. And you may also want to have a 'red line' where, if you get as high as that red line – no ifs, buts, or maybes – you have strayed and you must do something about it. We also considered a second red line, which was a weight you would not go *below* – probably not a concern for many people, but it does happen for some.

Especially in maintenance, we think it best to take a broad view and not to react too quickly to obvious natural weight fluctuations, such as those that can follow a weekend of celebrations. Maintainers, especially those who have been maintaining for quite some time, are likely to have acquired good dieting habits that will usually enable them to correct any short-term weight changes. But if you are now sure that you have strayed and that corrective action is needed, read on ...

### How did that straying happen?
Slice 26 is the corresponding slice to this one, covering getting back on track while losing weight. Some of the emphasis is different, but that is a good slice to re-read as a refresher.

The reason for straying in maintenance could be one (or more) of any number of old habits that you have slipped back into. If you realise which habits those are, you are better placed to know what you need to do to fix the situation and get back on track.

## How do you get back on track?
The principles of getting back on track, having strayed in maintenance, are exactly the same as when you strayed during weight loss and as we discussed in slice 26. As a quick reminder:

• Know how your straying happened (see a few lines above).

• Use the parts of this book relevant to your own particular reasons for straying.

• Be resourceful; use what we have written to problem-solve and find your own solutions.

If your reasons for straying were less well-defined (for example, 'I just couldn't be bothered anymore'), then, if you do not intend to give up entirely, we think the best idea is to have another look at slice 3, about motivation.

If *that* does not put you back on the right track, then we suggest that you go back to basics and work through the whole of the book again. We are not talking here about a quick skim read. Your weight-loss journey has involved a lot of hard work to get down to your target weight and then even more hard work to maintain that target weight, possibly for a long time. How could you now abandon all that you have achieved and slide back to being overweight? So we don't just ask, we *implore* you to go right back to the preamble (remember that?!) and start again. Follow the book 100 per cent – as if it were your first week!

We have never suggested that everything we have done ourselves to lose weight and maintain has been perfect. In fact, we think that it's because we have walked the (sometimes difficult) walk that we have been able to write a book that we hope will be useful to others. Certainly we have made mistakes, just like everyone else, so let's use our final chat time to give you examples of how our maintenance faltered and how we got back on track.

### CHAT TIME

*CAROLINE: Do you remember that difficult time we both went through in January a few years ago?*

*STEVE: Oh yes. It was pure coincidence, but we had similar experiences. And for a time we thought that we were going to be in big trouble with our weight.*

*CAROLINE: Yes, we did. I had been maintaining around the bottom of my acceptable weight band through most of the year, but I came out of the Christmas period a lot heavier than I went in. I did manage to lose some of that gain in January, and I still needed to lose more, but then my weight just stopped moving. Worst of all, I couldn't see why I wasn't losing any more. Things weren't good for you either, were they?*

*STEVE: No. In the autumn I had weighed rather more than I wanted – right at the top of my acceptable weight band. Before going away for Christmas I had used 'Ann's idea' [see slice 48] and managed to get down to the middle of my weight band. When I came back, Ann's idea had worked fine – but I was still only back to my autumn weight (in other words, too much).*

*CAROLINE: Still, that wasn't too bad, and Ann's idea had worked out well.*

*STEVE: True. But I did want to get to the middle of my acceptable weight band. So I really tried hard to lose more. When I try hard like that, I usually lose reasonably well, but this time I didn't. In fact, after losing just a little and then wobbling about for a time, my weight started to go up again. It was so high that it was getting near to my red-line weight [see slice 33 about red-line weights].*

*CAROLINE: We were similar – both of us couldn't get to the weight we thought was OK. We each had a worrying time, with the risk that it would turn into a major problem.*

*STEVE: Yes, it was clearly important to know what was causing the problem. But we didn't really know.*

*CAROLINE: That wasn't very clever of us. We didn't look too hard at what we were doing wrong, but we just kept on dieting as we always had before. Then we got lucky because the three of us (including Ann) were asked to write a joint blog about our recent dieting experiences.*

*STEVE: And that stirred things up. I think that you and I had* recently agreed to be one another's diet coach, and it inspired me to ask you whether we could share our online Nutracheck food diaries for three weeks. Those three weeks were the first time we had seen, in detail, what our daily calories consumed and burned were.

CAROLINE: It gave us a lot of interesting information, and I think we both looked with a renewed interest at our own eating habits.

STEVE: For my part, I saw how many calories I was drinking in the form of beer (too many, so I cut down), I began to record my daily steps (too few, so I increased them), and I made a lot of small permanent changes.

CAROLINE: Me too (except wine, not beer). And the result was that just over those three weeks, we got more or less to the weights we wanted to be – those target weights that we had struggled so much to achieve.

STEVE: And what was funny was that Ann had been taking part as well, just to give us some extra information about details of calories. She wasn't trying to lose weight, but she lost three pounds anyway!

CAROLINE: There was something else that I remember you found helpful – it was all to do with eating desserts in restaurants!

STEVE: Oh yes, that's true. When I was working away from home and eating in restaurants, I used to eat the sort of highly calorific desserts I would never touch at home. Then it struck me that that was a bit daft, and it motivated me not to eat such restaurant desserts in future. Even more than that, nowadays I seem to find motivation to change when I spot myself repeating something that's not helpful to my dieting ambitions.

CAROLINE: That might be a useful example for some. Maybe not many, but it's one more example of us all being different.

So what did we learn about getting back on track from the above experiences?

• When we were experiencing problems with our weight, we should have looked into what was causing the problems. If we had done that, we would not have lost our grip as worryingly as we did.

• The problems we found were not subtle or complicated. It was a clear case of weight control fatigue. We had slipped into habits of (1) consuming more high-calorie food (and drink), (2) increasing portion sizes, and (3) doing less exercise.

• There is a lot to be said for sharing experiences with others, including having a diet coach (see slices 11 and 37). In our case, we felt we were accountable to ourselves and we also felt some accountability to the thousands who would read the blog. We also found that a little hint of friendly competition was useful!

• Motivation can sometimes come in unexpected ways.

Things turned out well, and in a very short time we made great strides towards the maintenance weights that we wanted. But it's surprisingly easy to stray, even for people with a lot of dieting experience who think they know enough to write a book on the subject! Especially for maintainers, weight control fatigue is never far away, and we need to keep exercising constant vigilance.

We were lucky to have had the impetus of the blog we were asked to write – it encouraged us to look at what we had been doing wrong, so we could then problem-solve our way out of trouble. After a little stress, we realised that our whole straying experience had taught us something about our bodies and about keeping our weight under control. If you do stray and recover the situation, we do recommend that you try to learn from the experience as well. That learning will be useful if you stray again in the future.

# AND IN CONCLUSION

Way, way back at the very start of the book, we welcomed you
with a dramatic statement:

**Between the two of us, we lost fifteen stone, and we have kept it
off for several years. This book tells you how we did it,
and it will help you to do it too.**

We hope that we *have* helped you to do it – that you have arrived at your
target weight and that you have a good idea of how to maintain that
weight, not just for several years, but forever. We'd like to leave you with
three thoughts:

**Be constantly vigilant**

in particular

**Watch out for weight control fatigue**

and last but not least

**Don't forget to enjoy your food!**

# Acknowledgements

## By Steve

Quite soon after Caroline and I had a vague idea of writing something about maintaining a good weight loss forever, we realised what a huge task it was going to be. And *then* we realised what a variety of knowledge, experience, and skills would be needed. I thought that I had *some* of what was required for the task, but it was a constant delight (and relief) to find that what Caroline could bring to the table was remarkable. She has a rare ability to handle facts, figures, opinions, and tricky ideas and synthesise them into an interesting and insightful whole. But always with a sense of fun. She has simply been a joy to work with.

We have also had a great deal of help. Scattered throughout the book, there are more than fifty conversations, where we thought that a conversation was the best way of getting across the points we were making. We called those conversations 'chat times', and they were heavily based on talks or emails, which took place over a period of years.

Some chat times were between Caroline and myself, but many involved other people – people who gave us the benefit of their expertise and (sometimes painful) experiences of controlling their weight. We changed the names of the chat participants, usually because of the nature of the problems they shared with us. They generously gave us a lot of their time, and we can't thank them enough.

One person who is not anonymous is Ann, who is the kindest and most supportive wife in the world. She was hugely helpful in the project. It was Ann's suggestion that I join *Nutracheck*, and she was always there to encourage me on my weight-loss journey. Not only that, but she has been unswervingly enthusiastic about the book, even down to providing the first, fearless, and extremely useful editing of the manuscript. Thanks a million, chuck!

I would also like to acknowledge the contributions of the 'beta readers' Margaret Blake, Rachel Hartley, and Roz Watts. They read a late draft of the book, and each of them gave us a large number of invaluable suggestions for improvement.

After all of that editing and reviewing, the book was ready for professional editing, and I was fortunate to find a gem of an editor – Catherine Dunn. I firmly believed that our manuscript was spot-on, but Catherine quickly found and corrected a goodly number of errors, as well as finding countless ways of making the whole book more readable.

Finally, many thanks to Helen Hooker for her work on the cover of the book, including her double portrait of Caroline and myself.

## By Caroline

First and foremost, I'd like to thank Steve for suggesting that our ideas about losing weight and maintaining that loss deserved a wider audience and that we would fill more than a couple of sides of A4! The book would never have been written without the wonderful hospitality and friendship offered to me by Steve and Ann on our writing/walking weekends. Heartfelt thanks to them both for letting me share their lives for a while – and for so many delicious, inventive, and low-calorie meals. Steve took over the lion's share of the writing and editing when my workload increased – without that, the book would not be in your hands now.

I'd also like to thank *Nutracheck*, especially Rachel and Emma, for the opportunities they have offered us, as well as their support. I first read Steve's ideas in the regular blog posts he wrote for them and later wrote a few of my own. Many of my ideas were honed on the *Nutracheck* forum and I owe especial debt to 'GoFlyAKite', who cheered me on as I first wrote about aspects of losing weight – even before I met Steve.

Finally, thanks to Taunton library, who offered us a space to write together.

CPSIA information can be obtained
at www.ICGtesting.com
Printed in the USA
LVHW030633281220
675196LV00007BA/351